100

FACES OF
HEALTH CARE

100

FACES OF HEALTH CARE

AMERICAN HOSPITAL ASSOCIATION

HEALTH FORUM, INC.
An American Hospital Association Company
Chicago

Printed in the United States of America—3/99

Jacket/cover photo sources: (clockwise) Corbis-Bettmann (first five photos), *AHA News* archive, The History Museum for Springfield-Greene County

Jacket and cover design by Tim Kaage
Design and production coordination by Elm Street Publishing Services, Inc.

ISBN: 1-55648-276-0

Item Number: 070196

CONTENTS

FOREWORD

As the American Hospital Association prepared to celebrate its centennial year in 1998, the Centennial Planning Committee firmly believed that the celebration had two equally compelling roles: first, to show us how we have become who we are; and second, to set the vision for the future.

The articles and photographs which comprise *100 Faces of Health Care* initially appeared weekly in *AHA News* throughout the centennial year. They trace the history of health care in this nation through the people and events that shaped medicine and health care delivery. The photographs show the faces of health care providers—physicians, nurses, trustees, volunteers, and technicians—and the faces of their patients. They show the leaders in government and business who forged today's payment and coverage system. And while the images capture the overwhelming humanity of our profession, the words show us the challenges surmounted by hospitals and health care systems—the path traveled to where we are today.

100 Faces of Health Care celebrates the character, innovation, heroism, and dedication of those who created the profession of health care administration and who brought health care services to a developing nation. This book commemorates and celebrates the spirit that will shape health care for the coming century.

Gail L. Warden
Chairman
AHA Centennial Planning Committee

John G. King
1998 Chairman
AHA Board of Trustees

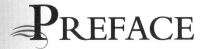PREFACE

The American Hospital Association (AHA) began with a handful of hospital leaders who met in Cleveland, Ohio, to exchange new ideas and information and to form the "Association of Hospital Superintendents." They chose as the association's mission: "To facilitate the interchange of ideas, comparing and contrasting methods of management, the discussion of hospital economics, the inspection of hospitals, suggestions of better plans for operating them, and such other matters as may affect the general interest of the membership."

It was a new era for hospitals, as they began their journey from "refuges for the destitute" (in the words of an early AHA chairman) to not only centers of technology and healing for all Americans but also essential cornerstones of every community in which they existed. The association grew in size, role, and stature, alongside the institutions it served.

Throughout 1998, the AHA celebrated its centennial—100 years of "health, caring, and unity"—with projects reaching out to all member hospitals and health care systems, state associations, regional/metropolitan associations, and personal membership groups.

In addition to the "100 Faces of Health Care" series in *AHA News* and the AHA history included in this book, the AHA's centennial was marked by a gala dinner at the 1998 AHA Annual Meeting, a video on the history of American hospitals, a traveling exhibit, and a Regional Leadership Forum held in Cleveland near the site where the association was founded. All of these projects and events were funded with the help of corporate sponsorships.

In these projects and events, the AHA's 1998 centennial recognized more than the life of an association. It spoke to the remarkable achievements of today's hospitals and health care systems and the value they continue to provide to their communities. It resonated with the message of what we can accomplish when working together.

On behalf of the American Hospital Association Board of Trustees, I am pleased to share with you this publication commemorating the history and accomplishments of hospitals, health care, and the American Hospital Association.

Dick Davidson
President
American Hospital Association

⪻Acknowledgments

AHA Centennial Planning Committee

Gail L. Warden, *chair, President and CEO of Henry Ford Health System, Detroit, MI, 1995 AHA chairman*

James Barber, *President of Healthcare Association of Southern California, Los Angeles, CA*

H. Robert Cathcart, *retired CEO of Pennsylvania Hospital, Philadelphia, PA, 1976 AHA chairman*

Joyce C. Clifford, R.N., *Vice President for Nursing of Beth Israel Hospital, Boston, MA, former AHA Board member*

Edward J. Connors, *President of Connors/Roberts & Associates, Morrisville, VT, 1989 AHA chairman*

James E. Dalton, Jr., *President and CEO of Quorum Health Group, Brentwood, TN*

Dick Davidson, *President of American Hospital Association, Washington, DC*

Anne Hall Davis, *Trustee of Cape Cod Hospital, Hyannis, MA, former AHA Board member*

Edward Eckenhoff, *President and CEO of National Rehabilitation Hospital, Washington, DC, former AHA Board member*

Yoshi Honkawa, *Consultant for Cedars-Sinai Medical Center, Los Angeles, CA, former chair AHAPAC*

John G. King, *CEO of Legacy Health System, Portland, OR, 1998 AHA chairman*

Carolyn Lewis, *Trustee of Greater Southeast Community Hospital, Washington, DC, 1999 AHA chairman-elect*

J. Alexander McMahon, *Executive-in-Residence of Fuqua School of Business, Duke University, Durham, NC, past AHA president*

Gary Mecklenburg, *President and CEO of Northwestern Memorial Hospital, Chicago, IL, AHA Board member*

Jack W. Owen, *former AHA Executive Vice President, Keswick, VA*

Lynn R. Olman, *President of Greater Cincinnati Hospital Council, Cincinnati, OH*

Carolyn C. Roberts, *President of Copley Health Systems, Inc., Morrisville, VT, 1994 AHA chair*

Stephen Rogness, *retired President of Minnesota Hospital and Healthcare Partnership, St. Paul, MN*

Ruth M. Rothstein, *Chief & Hospital Director of Cook County Bureau of Health Services, Cook County Hospital, Chicago, IL, AHA Board member*

Kenneth Rutledge, *President of Oregon Association of Hospitals and Health Systems, Lake Oswego, OR*

Amy Selene, *Des Moines, IA, past chair AHA Committee on Volunteers*

Staff: Michael P. Guerin, *Senior Vice President and Secretary of American Hospital Association*

The "100 Faces of Health Care" series, in its weekly appearances in *AHA News*, was made possible in part by educational grants from:

AHA Insurance Resource Inc.
PricewaterhouseCoopers
Merck & Co., Inc.
Medtronic
VALIC

The American Hospital Association's extensive centennial programs and projects would not have been possible without the Centennial Planning Committee, the members of which are listed to the left. The committee advised staff on projects, provided a historical perspective, and raised funds for the celebration. Gail L. Warden, committee chair and president and CEO of Henry Ford Health System in Detroit, provided guidance, enthusiasm, leadership, and a strong commitment to creating a meaningful celebration. John G. King, the AHA's centennial year chairman of the Board of Trustees and member of the Centennial Planning Committee, also gave his contagious and heartfelt support to the centennial celebration.

Special appreciation is due to Mary Grayson, editorial director of Health Forum, Inc., and Liz Oplatka, former editor of *AHA News*, who enthusiastically embraced the project and brought it from concept to weekly fruition. Laura Duggan, *AHA News* graphic designer, and Donald McGhie, former picture editor of *AHA News*, created the arresting appearance of the series through historic photos and article design. The AHA Resource Center provided valuable supporting materials. Many thanks to the staff of *AHA News* and AHA Press, who together helped to create *100 Faces of Health Care*. Michael Lesparre mined and refined the AHA's history into "A Century of the American Hospital Association." Michael P. Guerin, Gail M. Lovinger, Kathy Poole, and Ann Danns of the AHA's Office of the Secretary, Herman Baumann of the Health Research and Educational Trust, and Etta Fielek of the AHA's Communications Group all provided staff support for the Centennial Planning Committee.

AHA Insurance Resource Inc.

PRICEWATERHOUSE COOPERS 🔣

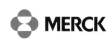 MERCK   Medtronic 🔲   VALIC

100

FACES OF
HEALTH CARE

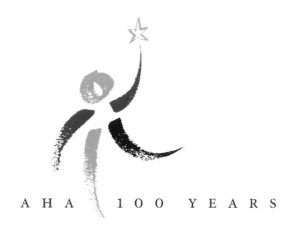

A H A   1 0 0   Y E A R S

INNOVATION IN A NATION DIVIDED

Civil War Battlefields Give Rise to Medical Advances

by Jon Asplund

War, with all its nightmarish suffering, has been an engine for innovation throughout the history of health care. The Civil War, like no war before, brought graphic newspaper depictions of that suffering to a horrified public on both sides, spurring an outcry for better care of the soldiers wounded right here on American soil.

Families "wanted to make sure their loved ones were well taken care of," said Gordon Dammann, founder and chairman of the National Museum of Civil War Medicine.

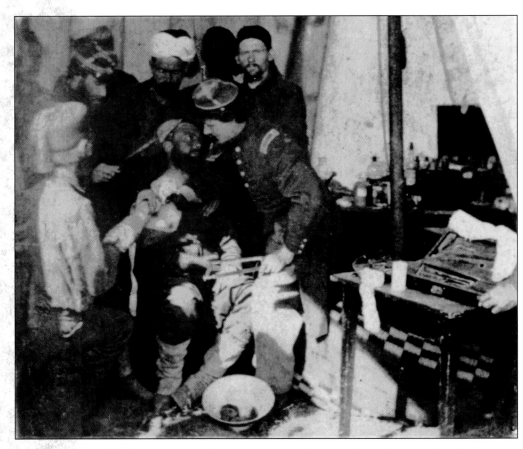

Field medicine, as this demonstration of amputation by soldiers in "Union Zouaves" uniforms shows, could be a gruesome, unsanitary task. But contrary to popularly held belief, anesthesia was used in 95 percent of medical procedures on soldiers wounded in the Civil War.

Photo courtesy of National Museum of Civil War Medicine, Frederick, MD.

Enter Dr. Jonathan Letterman

As medical director of the Union's Army of the Potomac, Letterman became "the father of American military medicine, bringing advances in field dressing and in the battleground evacuation procedure still known as the Letterman Plan," Dammann said.

Letterman pioneered the use of ambulances in the United States. The wounded men were evacuated from battlefields to field hospitals just a few miles behind the lines in "barns, farmhouses, schools, any place with shelter and water," Dammann said.

They were transferred later to hospitals in large cities. Many of those hospitals were makeshift setups in schools and government buildings with thousands of beds.

U.S. Surgeon General William Hammond gave Letterman *carte blanche* to organize his ambulance system, and helped Letterman codify his mobile hospital organization in the 1864 "Act to Establish a Uniform System of Ambulances in the Armies of the United States."

Medical Mythology

"Misconceptions abound about Civil War medicine," Dammann said.

Amputation was a common remedy for gunshot wounds to the arms and legs, but not because surgeons in the mid-19th century were barbaric "sawbones" with little understanding of how to save the limbs of injured soldiers.

Most Civil War wounds came from Minie balls—.58-caliber, soft-lead bullets that would flatten out on impact, shattering and splintering flesh and bone.

The violence of such wounds, compounded with unsanitary conditions on the battlefield, made infection a major threat, Dammann said. Amputation to halt the spread of infection actually saved many soldiers' lives.

More than 620,000 people perished in the Civil War, two-thirds of them from disease, pointed out Laura Mumm, public relations and marketing coordinator for the Civil War Medicine Museum.

Another misconception is that primitive medicine and a lack of supplies meant the only way most soldiers could deal with excruciating pain was to "bite the bullet."

On the contrary, Mumm said, anesthetics were used in 95 percent of procedures, even in the Confederacy, which had much fewer supplies than the Union as the war progressed.

Ether or chloroform was used during operations, and a variety of painkillers, mainly morphine derivatives, were used to ease pain afterward.

The heavy use of such anesthetics greatly contributed to medicine's understanding of them, Dammann said.

The New Hospital

Physicians' experiences during the Civil War also led to practices that presaged the "germ theory" that would later lead physicians to understand the importance of cleanliness, Dammann said.

Soldiers often fared better in field hospitals than in regular hospitals, leading to the "ventilation theory" that regards sunlight, clean air and clean sheets as important aids in recovery.

"Before that, it was assumed that the night air contained noxious vapors, and all the drapes and windows were closed," creating a breeding ground for disease, Dammann said.

A Woman's Place

Prior to the Civil War, hospitals were a male domain, even when it came to nurses. Women tended to the sick only in their own homes or, as midwives, in other homes.

But able-bodied male nurses joined the army once war was declared, and women were pressed into service on the homefront.

"They took a lot of heat from physicians and surgeons," Dammann said. "But some of the first women to work in hospitals were Catholic sisters, and they were seen as above the gender problem. The surgeons finally had to cave in.

"The soldiers all referred to their nurses as 'mother' and they were the ones who held the soldiers' hands as they took their last breath."

Dammann, a Lena, IL, dentist, founded the National Museum of Civil War Medicine in Frederick, MD, last spring after more than 21 years of collecting some 3,000 Civil War-era medical items, including surgeons' tents, uniforms and medical devices. For information, call the National Museum of Civil War Medicine at (301) 695-1864.

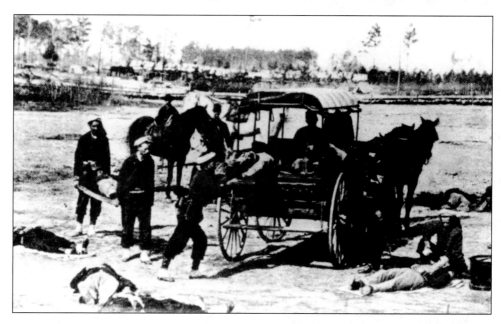

Soldiers participate in an ambulance drill by the Union's Army of the Potomac in 1864. Speed and safety were of utmost importance in saving soldiers wounded on the battlefield, leading to the creation of a modern, organized ambulance corps.

Photo courtesy of National Museum of Civil War Medicine, Frederick, MD.

WHERE THE EVOLUTION BEGAN

Colonial Doctor Gives American Hospitals a Revolutionary Beginning

by Philip Dunn

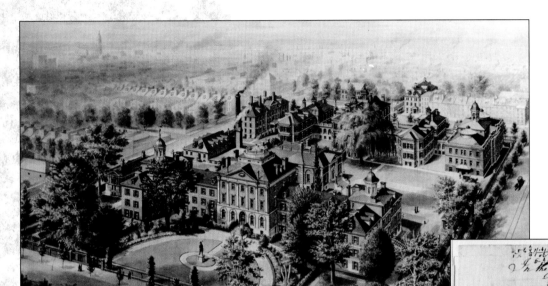

Above, an artist's conception of a bird's-eye view of Pennsylvania Hospital as it looked at the turn of the century in Philadelphia's historic Society Hill. Right, Benjamin Franklin's original manuscript of the inscription of the cornerstone of the hospital's east wing, laid May 28, 1755.

Photos provided by Pennsylvania Hospital.

In 1750, Thomas Bond, a European-trained physician, developed the harebrained notion to establish a hospital in his native Philadelphia. Like a lot of other pie-in-the-sky ideas floating around the colonies, Bond's proposal went nowhere.

Bond couldn't sell the idea because most people who could afford it received care in their homes. Although a voluntary hospital movement was building in Europe, it just didn't seem necessary in the colonies.

Then Bond enlisted the help of a friend named Benjamin Franklin.

Franklin, the scientist, inventor and publisher (and future revolutionary) used his ties to the business and political elite of the fledgling city to raise enough money

and confidence to get Pennsylvania Hospital, the nation's first inpatient hospital, off the ground.

With just a few months of lobbying, Franklin managed to get 33 city leaders to sign a petition, which was presented to the Pennsylvania Assembly on Jan. 20, 1751, according to William H. Williams' history of the hospital, *America's First Hospital: The Pennsylvania Hospital, 1751–1841.* The goal, according to the petition, was to help the so-called "sick-poor"—to aid "such, whose poverty is made more miserable by the additional weight of grievous disease from which they might easily be relieved."

On May 11, 1751, the Assembly granted Pennsylvania Hospital a charter. In extracting that support, Franklin, ever the inventor, devised a new fund-raising technique—

the matching fund drive—when the Assembly promised to contribute 2,000 pounds sterling toward the effort only if hospital organizers could come up with an equal amount.

First Among Equals

From the start, Pennsylvania Hospital faced challenges that are no doubt familiar to hospital administrators even today—raising capital, generating popular support and defining its mission.

With Pennsylvania's urbanization, it became clear that to send the ill "industrious poor" back to their home villages would cost too much. Similar thinking spurred the European voluntary hospital movement.

"Franklin's thesis [was] that an organized group of men working for a common goal can do more good in the world than if each man worked to help his neighbors by himself," wrote I. Bernard Cohen in his introduction of a reprint of Franklin's early history of the hospital.

But unlike Europe's voluntary hospitals, Pennsylvania Hospital's founders agreed the facility should admit paying patients when there was room. In that sense, the Philadelphia hospital was an innovator.

Pennsylvania Hospital broke ground in other ways:

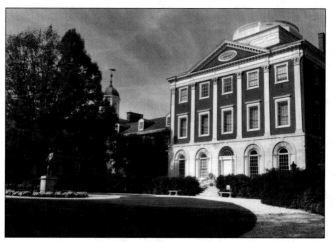

The hospital's Pine Building today houses the medical library and the surgical amphitheater.

Photo provided by Pennsylvania Hospital.

- In 1762, a British friend of Franklin, Dr. John Fothergill, donated a book to what became the nation's first medical library at the hospital. In 1847, the American Medical Association designated it as the first, largest and most important medical library in the United States.
- In 1773, 16-year-old Jacob Ehrenzeller Jr., son of a local tavern owner, was appointed the hospital's first medical resident. In his five-year internship, Ehrenzeller was to combine clinical training at the hospital with education at the College of Philadelphia (another institution founded by Franklin, later renamed the University of Pennsylvania).

Unfortunately, the Revolutionary War forced the college to close temporarily, and Ehrenzeller never received his degree. Still, he was one of the first doctors able to support his family solely on income earned practicing medicine.

- In 1794, Dr. Phillip Syng Physick, known as the "father of American surgery," was appointed to the hospital's medical staff. In 1812, Physick introduced the stomach pump.
- In 1804, the nation's first surgical amphitheater was constructed.
- In 1812, Dr. Benjamin Rush, who had been on the medical staff of Pennsylvania Hospital for nearly 30 years, published the nation's first psychiatric textbook, *Observations and Inquiries Upon the Diseases of the Mind.* Rush, a signer of the Declaration of Independence, is known as the "father of American psychiatry."

Other Pennsylvania Hospital firsts include the introduction of occupational therapy (1752), the first description of hemophilia (1834), the first hospital care of mentally ill patients (1752) and the first daily record of weather conditions (1766).

Today, Pennsylvania Hospital is a 739-bed institution, with a 505-bed facility in Philadelphia's Society Hill and a 234-bed psychiatric hospital in West Philadelphia. It performs about 15,000 surgeries a year, including 1,800 joint replacements—the most in the nation.

But the hospital has not escaped the realities of the modern health care marketplace. In 1997, for the first time in its history, the hospital affiliated with another institution, joining with the University of Pennsylvania Health System.

One thing that has not changed is the cornerstone, written by Franklin, which still stands at the hospital's Pine Building. It reads:

In the year of Christ MDCCLV
George the Second happily reigning
(for he sought the happiness of his people)
Philadelphia flourishing
(for its inhabitants were publick spirited)
this building
by the bounty of the government,
and of many private persons,
was piously founded
for the relief of the sick and miserable;
may the God of mercies
bless the undertaking

WHO YOU GONNA CALL?

Not Long Ago, a Trip by Ambulance Could Be a Wild Ride

by Kevin Murray

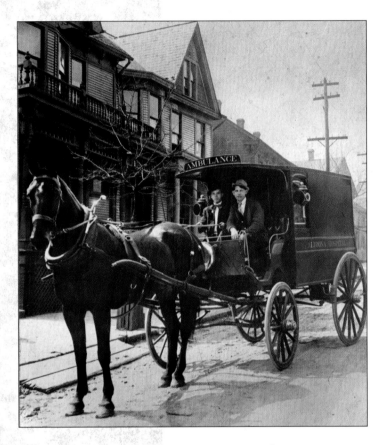

A horse-drawn ambulance waits to transport a patient in Altoona, PA, in 1906. As late as the 1960s, funeral homes provided the only ambulance service for many communities.

Source: AHA News archive

Imagine you are driving down the road in the early 1960s when suddenly you crash head-on with another car. You remain conscious long enough to realize that you have been extricated from the car and placed in the back of a hearse.

Thirty-five years ago, funeral homes provided ambulance service in many parts of the country.

"They typically were the only ones with vehicles long enough where you could lie someone down," says Dan Manz, immediate past president of the Falls Church, VA-based National Association of State Emergency Medical Services Directors. "In addition to a public-relations vehicle, the funeral homes viewed ambulance services as a feeder mechanism" for their businesses.

Back then, few cities provided much in the way of emergency services, he says, and there was little research into the science of emergency care as compared with other areas of medicine. Manz attributes that apathy to society's fatalistic approach toward traumatic injuries.

"We had grown accustomed to the idea of 'Old Joe' goes out, smacks his car into a tree and gets hurt real bad. He's either going to die or get better—one of the two," he says. "There isn't a whole lot that emergency care is going to do to alter the path that Old Joe goes down."

Turning Point

Perhaps the most significant development in the evolution of EMS was the 1966 publication of a "white paper" by the National Academy of Science. "Accidental Death and Disability: The Neglected Disease of Modern Society" outlined how improved EMS—including more competent initial emergency medical care, more efficient transportation and more active treatment—could dramatically reduce the high percentage of deaths and disabilities from automobile accidents.

Following the release of the document, Congress passed the Highway Safety Act of 1966, which set up the federal Department of Transportation (DOT). The act stipulated that the secretary of transportation is responsible for reducing motor vehicle deaths and injuries by setting standards, including one establishing EMS training programs for all people who provide care to those injured on the highways.

"At that time, the extent of the [EMS] training basically was the advanced first-aid training you could get from the American Red Cross," says David Nevins, executive vice president of the Sacramento, CA-based American Ambulance Association.

Nevins points out that advanced EMS training was of no practical use because ambulance services only responded to an accident, picked up the patients and transported them to the hospital.

Many hospitals were ill-prepared to receive trauma patients.

"Hospitals were closing the doors of their emergency departments at 11 p.m., and staffing in the emergency room often was seen [by hospital staff] as penalty duty," Manz says.

In the late 1960s, the DOT commissioned a panel of experts—including physicians, funeral home directors, fire chiefs who were running model programs, and officials of the American Red Cross—to identify the knowledge, skills, practical abilities and equipment that people riding in ambulances needed. The panel concluded that EMS personnel needed to know how to open an airway, perform CPR, control bleeding, and deliver a baby. Necessary equipment included cervical collars, oxygen systems, backboards, bandaging materials, splints and obstetrical kits.

Once better-trained personnel were employed on ambulances, they clamored for better equipment and vehicles.

Nevins points to the three-digit emergency-response telephone number (911) as one of the biggest breakthroughs in the emergency medical services field. It started on a limited basis in the early 1960s, but soon gained wide public acceptance. "Everyone knows, even from very small children, to pick up the phone [and dial 911] if they perceive to have an emergency, whether it's medical, police or fire," he says.

By the early 1970s, most states had instituted training programs for emergency medical technicians (EMTs) and paramedics. As more people became EMTs and paramedics, the EMS systems started evolving in the early-to mid-1970s, beginning with the first response and ambulance transport systems.

Just Like on TV

Emergency, a 1970s television show that featured two Los Angeles paramedics traveling the streets in an ambulance and saving lives, significantly increased public awareness of EMS, Nevins says.

"Suddenly, people throughout the country are watching this program and saying, 'Why don't we have guys like this?' " he said.

Training of EMS personnel increased during the 1980s as medical techniques improved and procedures that traditionally were performed in a hospital environment were being performed in a pre-hospital setting.

"Instead of being transported to the hospital to properly diagnose and treat patients' injuries, the medical equipment now comes to the patient," Nevins said.

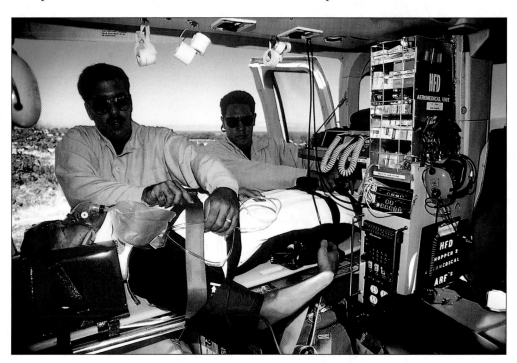

An emergency medical services crew tends to an injured patient during an air ambulance rescue in Hawaii in 1995. Today, highly skilled ambulance teams using the latest medical equipment can perform sophisticated lifesaving procedures before patients even reach the hospital.

Source: G. Brad Lewis/Tony Stone Images Inc.

POLITICS, PATIENCE AND FINALLY MEDICARE

A Long and Bumpy Road Leads to a Historic Signing in Independence, MO

by Alwyn Cassil

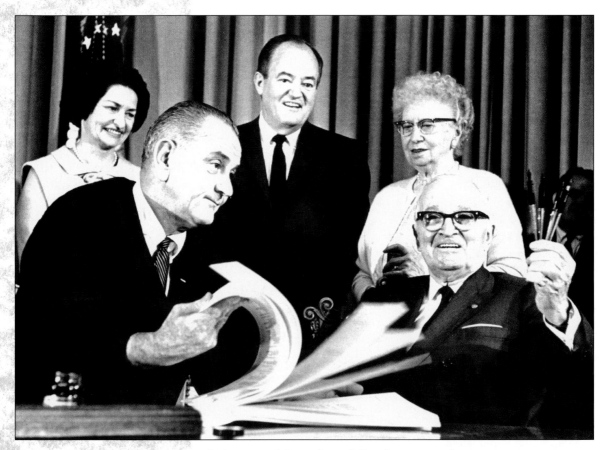

President Lyndon Johnson flips through the pages of the Medicare bill as former President Harry Truman triumphantly waves the pens that will be used to sign the legislation into law. Johnson brought the signing ceremony to Independence, MO, on July 30, 1965, to share the spotlight with Truman, who had unsuccessfully proposed a national health insurance plan two decades before. Looking on are Lady Bird Johnson, Vice President Hubert Humphrey and Bess Truman. Source: Corbis-Bettmann/UPI

The mood was jubilant as Air Force One and a second plane carried President Lyndon Johnson and his entourage on a pilgrimage to Independence, MO, hometown of Harry Truman.

The day was July 30, 1965, and that afternoon as about 200 people watched the making of history in the tiny Truman Library, Johnson signed the Medicare bill into law.

With a stroke of his pen—actually, he used 72 pens to sign the legislation—Johnson laid a cornerstone of his promised Great Society.

"It was typical Johnson to fly us all down to Independence," recalled former Social Security Commissioner Robert Ball, who oversaw making the Medicare law into a working national hospital insurance program for almost 20 million Americans 65 and older. Johnson had a flair for the dramatic, according to Ball.

Medicare's lineage led straight back to Truman, who nearly two decades before had unsuccessfully proposed a national health insurance plan for all Americans. Many people had championed Medicare over the years, Johnson noted, "But it all really started with the man from Independence, and so as it should be, we've come back here to his home to complete what he began."

The 81-year-old Truman said, "I am glad to have lived this long and to witness the signing of the Medicare bill."

If the American Medical Association (AMA) had had its way, Truman would never have had seen Medicare become a reality. As far back as 1945 when Truman first proposed universal coverage, the AMA adamantly opposed government involvement in medicine.

After the 1964 presidential election and Johnson's landslide victory, the question became not if Medicare would pass but when.

Following Johnson's call for action on Medicare in his 1965 State of the Union address, Democratic leaders in both houses arranged for identical bills to be introduced by Sen. Clinton P. Anderson of New Mexico and Rep. Cecil R. King of California. The bill had passed the Senate but not the House in the previous session when the measure couldn't get past Rep. Wilbur Mills, the Arkansas Democrat who ruled the Ways and Means Committee.

After the election, Mills realized that Medicare in some form was inevitable. Ever the consummate politician, he decided the best defense was a good offense and made the legislation his own.

Mills knew that the King-Anderson bill would fall sorely short of the public's expectations—a Gallup poll

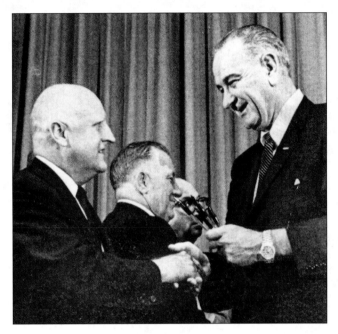

Kenneth Williamson, director of the AHA Washington Service Bureau, shakes hands with Johnson following the signing. Despite opposition from the American Medical Association and others, Medicare became reality in part through expert political maneuvering by Rep. Wilbur Mills, himself a one-time opponent of the bill.

Source: AHA archive

in January 1965 showed that while two-thirds of Americans supported Medicare, 40 percent believed it would cover all medical expenses.

At about the same time, the AMA fought Medicare by claiming its coverage was inadequate. The doctors came up with their own plan, dubbed Eldercare, that would build on the 1960 Kerr-Mills law providing federal matching money to states for elderly people who weren't on welfare but couldn't pay their own medical bills. Few states had taken advantage of Kerr-Mills. Not to be left out, the Republicans introduced Bettercare, which would subsidize the voluntary purchase of comprehensive private health insurance for the elderly, depending on income.

In early March, as the Ways and Means Committee prepared to take up the Medicare bill, Mills called on Wilbur Cohen, an assistant secretary of the Department of Health, Education and Welfare, to provide an overview of the bills. Cohen later described what happened next as the "most brilliant legislative move I'd seen in 30 years."

Mills decided to turn Medicare, Bettercare and Eldercare into one "three-layer cake." The Eldercare layer, which would later be known as Medicaid, would provide care for the poor; the Medicare layer would cover hospital, nursing and home-health care for the rest of the elderly; and the voluntary Bettercare layer would cover doctors' bills, both in and out of the hospital, if people paid a small monthly premium.

"In effect, Mills had taken the AMA's ammunition, put it in the Republicans' gun, and blown both of them off the map," Cohen observed later.

Mills' package would face more assaults, but in the end, both the House and Senate passed the bill by overwhelming margins.

RECONCILING ROLES

*A Century after Achieving Professional Legitimacy,
Nurses Still Struggle with Image*

by Matthew Weinstock

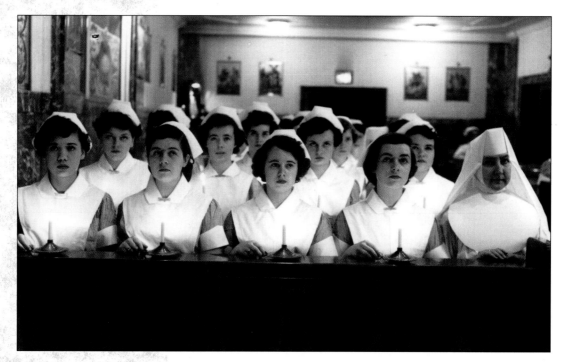

*Freshmen receive their caps at a hospital nursing school ceremony in 1954. They hold lights symbolic of
the lamp carried by Florence Nightingale. After World War II, more nurses received vigorous scientific
training but continued to encounter sexist attitudes about their profession.*   Source: Corbis-Bettmann

Nurses have been classified by a series of conflict-ing images: autonomous practitioner vs. sub-servient employee, angel of mercy vs. clinician. These images started to clash in the late 19th century. Until then, nurses were viewed primarily as guardian angels and doctors' handmaidens.

In the latter half of the century, however, nursing had an awakening of sorts. Training schools sprung up nation-wide. Florence Nightingale and other nursing leaders used science to re-create society's understanding of nurses and nursing, said Joan Lynaugh, professor emeri-tus of the University of Pennsylvania and former director of the school's Center for the Study of the History of Nursing.

As a result, nurses gained greater influence in hospi-tals. No longer merely custodians, they used their training to make hospitals safer, healthier places.

For example, nurses linked poor sanitary conditions to increased mortality rates. They understood that freshly laundered linens and improved ventilation would improve care for the ill.

In June 1893, the world stood witness as these conflict-ing images collided. It occurred at the Columbian Exposition, commonly referred to as the Chicago World's Fair, one of the most spectacular international gatherings of its time. The latest and greatest technologies were on exhibit—Pullman cars, structural steel and the first Ferris wheel.

It also is considered by many as one of the most signifi-cant events in the history of nursing. Isabel Stewart, one of the era's nursing leaders, proclaimed it the "coming-out party of nursing as a profession."

At the fair, nursing leaders called on their peers to become more vigilant in promoting health standards.

A paper written by Nightingale urged nurses to go into their communities and become "health missioners," to visit families in their homes and talk about healthy living.

The Chicago fair also marked the rise of the first professional nursing organizations, the Society of Superintendents of Training Schools for Nurses and the Nursing Associated Alumnae, which became the American Nurses Association (ANA) in 1911. Both promoted nursing as a legitimate profession and fought for better working conditions for nurses, established codes of ethics and standardized training programs.

A Tough Fight

Still, it took decades for the public and other health professionals to recognize the importance of nursing as a profession, Lynaugh said, especially because sexism was still rampant.

In a 1908 article in the *New York Journal of Medicine*, a physician wrote that any "intelligent, not necessarily educated woman can in short time acquire the skill to carry out with implicit obedience the physician's direction."

Throughout the middle part of the 20th century, most people thought nurses simply did what doctors told them to do.

But behind the scenes, nurses were busy taking control of their destiny. After World War II, nursing leaders sought to establish more rigorous and more scientific training programs. As a result, a growing number of nurses started to receive their training from universities, rather than hospital-based schools.

"At hospital schools, science training was close to zip," Lynaugh said. "At university schools, the training was more intense. Nursing leaders pushed this educational reform after the war."

Nurses from New York City's Henry Street Settlement House set out for the homes of the poor in lower Manhattan in the early 1900s. At the Chicago World's Fair in 1893, Florence Nightingale called on her nursing peers to become 'health missioners' by going into communities to talk about healthy living.

Source: Corbis-Bettmann

Nonetheless, it was not until the social upheavals of the 1960s that nurses truly started to break new ground. "Nurse midwives, critical care nurses and nurse practitioners—registered nurses with advanced degrees—helped bring nursing out of the shadows," Lynaugh said.

"The creation of nurse practitioners (in the mid-1960s) created a whole new understanding of nurses," she said.

Old Meets New

That understanding was recognized in 1997 when a group of nurses established their own health care practice in New York City and were accredited as primary care providers by several insurance companies.

It was the first time nurse practitioners have been recognized officially as primary care providers.

"We can do some profound work," said Edwidge Thomas, a cofounder of the Columbia Advanced Practice Nurse Association. "Roles are changing in terms of what nurses can do and we are proof of that.

"We do not want to get rid of the angel of mercy image," she added. "We still want to care for you, but there is also a lot of scientific basis for what we do."

But it is those conflicting images that continue to plague nursing, according to Alison Kitson, a professor at the National Institute for Nursing at Oxford University in England.

We "have not united on the central image . . . that we want to communicate to the public," she argued in a speech last summer. We "still have not reconciled the dialectic tension between the scientific base of nursing and its moral base of care," she said.

THE FORGOTTEN PANDEMIC

Spanish Flu of 1918 Was Gravest Crisis American Hospitals Had Ever Faced

by Susannah Zak Figura

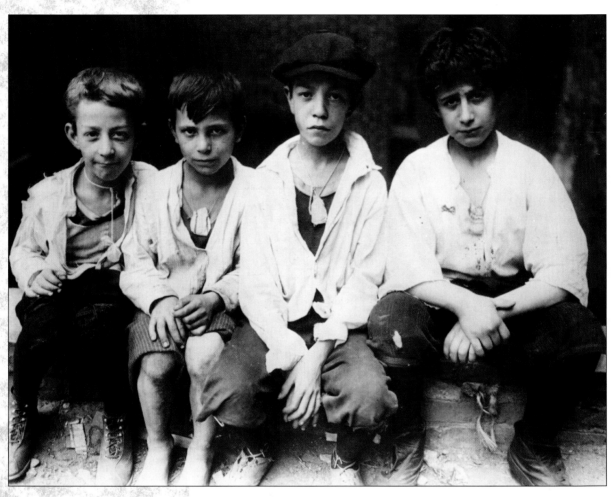

Some parents in 1918 made their children wear bags of camphor around their necks in the hope that it would ward off the Spanish Flu. The flu spread so quickly and struck so cruelly that children often collapsed in their classrooms.

Source: Corbis-Bettmann

Epidemiologists, virologists and public-health experts have been on top of the "Hong Kong Flu" outbreak practically since the first death last May. Eighty years ago, when the "Spanish Flu" whipped around the globe in three vicious stages, reaction was neither as swift nor as sophisticated.

More than 30 million people worldwide—550,000 in the United States—died from influenza and related pneumonia. For American hospitals, caring for the sick stretched resources in a way never experienced before.

"The 1918 crisis was the greatest yet faced by American hospitals," said Alfred Crosby, professor of history, American studies and geography at the University of Texas in Austin and author of *America's Forgotten Pandemic: The Influenza of 1918.*

"The cholera, typhoid and other epidemics of the 19th century were very bad," Crosby said. "But hospitals were smaller, the epidemics usually more localized . . . and people expected less of [hospitals]. Hospitals were where you went to die."

The three waves of flu that hit the United States between March 1918 and early 1919 traveled swiftly. It took only five months for the first wave to circle the globe.

Influenza expert W.I.B. Beveridge, author of *Influenza: The Last Great Plague*, recalled as a boy seeing classmates collapse suddenly from the sickness.

While the pandemic may have started in the United States, the virus was especially deadly in Spain, where it got lots of publicity and picked up its name.

Most people who contracted the virus recovered in a few days. But about 20 percent succumbed to pneumonia, according to Beveridge.

Of those who died, most were age 20 to 40.

"So many young adults died because they had healthy, vigorous immune systems, which over-reacted to the totally unfamiliar flu . . . flooding the lungs and drowning the sick," Crosby said.

Coping at Home

With many American physicians and nurses overseas on war duty, the nation was woefully unprepared. The few available health care workers, including some called out of retirement, barely kept up with demand. One San Jose, CA, physician saw 525 influenza patients in a single day.

Antibiotics were not yet available, so little could be done for the sick. In some cities, people died faster than coffins could be built and graves dug.

Still, hundreds of thousands of people at all levels of society volunteered to help where they could. Eleanor Roosevelt, for example, regularly took food to patients at a Red Cross hospital.

"To an amazing extent, enthusiasm was successfully substituted for preparation and efficiency in the battle with flu," Crosby said.

Local officials nationwide did their part to help stem the virus' spread.

In Chicago, Health Commissioner John Dill Robertson posted signs in movie houses declaring, "IF YOU HAVE A COLD AND ARE COUGHING AND SNEEZING DO NOT ENTER THIS THEATRE. GO HOME AND GO TO BED UNTIL YOU ARE WELL."

As conditions worsened, schools, theaters, churches and other public gathering sites closed down.

Philadelphia suffered most of major American cities, with the numbers of dead rising exponentially each week.

Hospital Challenges

Philadelphia hospitals soon burst at their seams, and emergency hospitals sprang up in parish houses and state armories. These extra facilities strained the already sparse health care force.

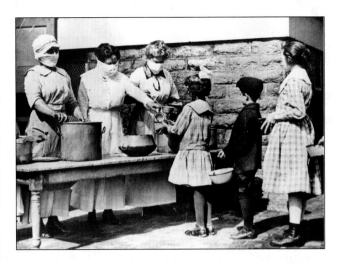

Volunteer workers wearing gauze masks serve a meal to the children of stricken parents in Cincinnati. Antibiotics were not yet available in 1918, and in some cities, coffin-makers and grave-diggers could not keep up with the casualties.

Source: Corbis-Bettmann

Pennsylvania Hospital had sent 75 percent of its medical and surgical staff overseas for the war effort. Many of those who remained fell with the flu. On one day, Philadelphia General Hospital had 52 nurses sick. Nearby Lebanon (PA) Hospital barely managed with three nurses for 125 flu victims.

To help prevent the flood of patients from overwhelming hospitals, city officials created seven districts with assigned medical staff and resources. Hospitals reported all discharges, whether of cured patients or dead ones, to district police, who saw that beds were immediately filled.

On the West Coast, despite fair warning that influenza was on its way, San Franciscans also were hit hard.

City officials put in place an ordinance requiring every "person appearing on the public streets, in any public place" to wear a mask.

As in Philadelphia, they divided the city into districts and apportioned medical resources.

San Francisco Hospital, designated as the isolation hospital for influenza victims, came close to collapse. About 78 percent of the hospital's nurses got influenza.

Surprisingly, the 1918 influenza did little to spur public-health efforts to avoid future epidemics, according to Edwin D. Kilbourne, research professor of microbiology and immunology at New York Medical College, Valhalla, NY.

Once the pandemic died down, people largely forgot about its devastating impact, he said. As Crosby puts it, the Spanish Flu of 1918 became the "forgotten pandemic."

BIRTH OF THE BLUES

American Health Insurance Began as an Effort to Save One Hospital

by Jon Asplund

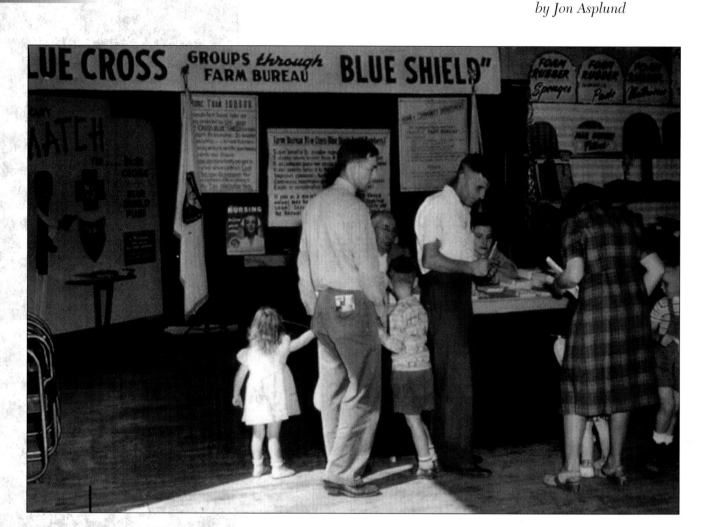

John Mannix, who helped establish the Cleveland Hospital Service Association, predicted at the 1929 AHA annual meeting that prepaid health plans would lead to an enormous increase in hospitalization demand. The plans grew phenomenally during the Depression through the post-World War II boom years. The Farm Bureau and other organizations helped promote the plans.

Source: Blue Cross Blue Shield Association archives

There's unprecedented economic growth and a stock market boom. There's nagging financial turmoil overseas. Health care operating costs are rising, hospital occupancy rates are falling, and the public is worried it won't be able to afford decent care.

Against that backdrop, a hospital administrator launches a program to finance hospital care, not just deliver it.

Sound like a blueprint for a modern provider-sponsored organization? Actually, it's how American health insurance was invented 70 years ago.

In 1929, Dallas schools Superintendent Justin Ford Kimball went to work for Baylor University. He had no knowledge of health care, but solid experience in administration and financial management, and he was charged with turning around the ailing University Hospital.

Under Kimball's direction, Baylor signed up Dallas schoolteachers for 50 cents a month each. That money went into a fund for the prepayment of the teachers' hospital care, according to *The Blues: A History of the Blue*

Cross and Blue Shield System put out last year by the Blue Cross and Blue Shield Association.

Prior to Kimball's brainchild, some industries' provided sick benefits and company doctors to their employees, but there had never been a real prepaid health care program in the United States.

Kimball's idea spread quickly and multihospital insurance plans began sprouting up under such names as the Hospital Care Association, in Durham, NC; Group Hospitalization, Washington, DC; and the Cleveland Hospital Service Association.

Those plans, formed separately but not independently of each other, began using a common symbol—a blue cross, according to Robert Cunningham III and Robert M. Cunningham Jr., who authored the Blues' history. The symbol, in turn, led to the common name.

Changes for Hospitals

The concept of prepaid health care posed dilemmas for providers.

John Robert Mannix, who helped set up the Cleveland plan, said at the AHA's 1929 annual meeting that insurance would change things, but if successful also would provide the funds to deal with those changes.

"You are going to have a great increase in the hospitalization demand," Mannix is quoted in "The Blues" as telling those attending the AHA meeting. "Many more people are going to come for illness and observation [who] don't come to the hospital . . . at present. For example, less than half the women having babies come to hospitals for maternity care; but if this plan were in effect, all those who have the insurance would come."

Doctors soon followed Kimball's lead, establishing the first "Blue Shield" plans for patients to prepay doctors' bills during the Great Depression.

The prepaid plans guaranteed both hospitals and doctors a source of income in uncertain times.

Boom Time

By guaranteeing health care to subscribers, the plans experienced extraordinary growth amid the hardships of

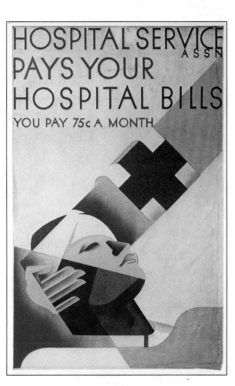

This poster, commissioned in 1934 initially for use by the Hospital Service Association, featured a blue cross, which has become one of the most recognizable and enduring symbols in trademark history. The Hospital Service Association later became Blue Cross of Minnesota.

Source: Blue Cross and Blue Shield of Minnesota

the 1930s, the mobilization for war in the 1940s and the postwar boom years.

The success came as a surprise to many doubters of prepaid health insurance.

In Lewis E. Weeks' hospital adminsitration oral history series, sponsored by the AHA, Mannix remembered "when we finally started the prepayment plan in Cleveland, Guy Clark, who was the executive of the [local] hospital council, bet me a straw hat we would not enroll 10,000 people in the plan within five years. We did that in less than a year."

He said that as recently as 1940, people had no idea how large Blue Cross would become.

"There were articles saying that while voluntary prepayment for care was a good idea, you could never expect to reach more than a small percentage of the population," Mannix said.

During World War II "growth was phenomenal. Although troop mobilizations drained membership ranks in some areas, war industries drew hundreds of thousands of new potential subscribers into the labor force," according to the Cunninghams, noting that "between 1939 and 1944, unemployment dropped from 17.2 to 1.2 percent."

The Blues used a variety of promotions to bring people into their plans.

The Hospital Service Association of Pittsburgh, which would later become Blue Cross of Western Pennsylvania, launched a public relations campaign featuring a series of cartoons. United Way organizations and Community Chest groups helped to get the uninsured into plans during once-a-year enrollment periods.

Although for-profit and other not-for-profit insurers started to get into the medical services arena, the Blues dominated the field.

They remain influential, with Blue Cross and Blue Shield logos among the most recognized trademarks, ranking right up there with McDonald's Golden Arches.

BANKROLLING BREAKTHROUGHS

National Institutes of Health Grants Transform American Medicine

by Susannah Zak Figura

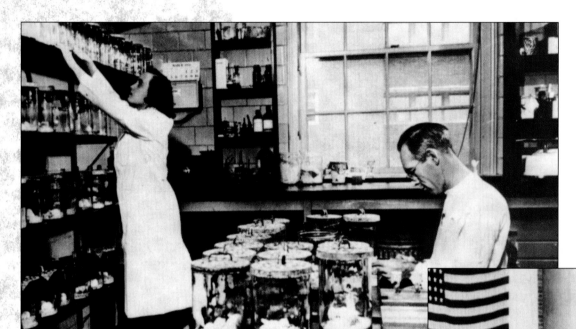

Above: Researchers at the National Institutes of Health conduct lab work in the 1940s. Americans had seen how sulfa drugs and pencillin helped soldiers wounded in World War II, and they pushed for more medical research.

Source: Corbis-Bettmann

Right: President Franklin D. Roosevelt dedicates the administration building on the NIH's new Bethesda headquarters in 1940.

Source: Corbis-Bettmann

A lot can happen in 50 years, and few know that better than America's teaching hospitals. Today, there are about 400 teaching hospitals nationwide. About 120 are part of academic medical centers, which include medical schools.

At this elite subset of institutions, the complex and fruitful marriage of scientific innovation, clinical know-how and financial support transforms ideas into cures.

These are the places where livers are transplanted, heart valves repaired and bone marrow replenished. These are the places where years are added to human lives.

Without research funding from the National Institutes of Health (NIH), experts say, these advances might never have been made, or would have taken a lot longer.

Before NIH grants, medical research was conducted "on an infinitesimally smaller scale," said David Korn, senior vice president of biomedical research at the Association of American Medical Colleges.

"The birth of the NIH as a major source of . . . research funding had an absolutely profound effect on medical schools and also on their teaching hospital partners," Korn said.

How It Began

The NIH has been around in concept since the late 19th century when the Hygienic Laboratory, part of the Staten Island (NY) Marine Hospital, examined sea passengers suspected of having infectious diseases.

The world's first laboratory diagnosis of cholera in the Western Hemisphere took place there in 1887.

In 1930, the Hygienic Laboratory officially became the National Institute of Health and in 1938 began the move to its current home in Bethesda, MD.

After individual research branches such as the National Cancer Institute and the National Heart Institute were created some years later, the entity came to be known as the National Institutes of Health.

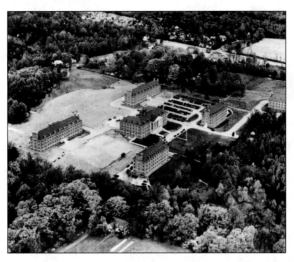

A view of the NIH campus in the 1940s, an era when the federal government was eager to pump research dollars through the NIH to nongovernment laboratories. The scientists' fear that anyone accepting such money would be corrupted led to a peer-review process for judging the merits of research proposals. That, in turn, has been called the "genius of the NIH" by experts because it creates competition, which "fosters creativity and raises the level of excellence." Source: National Institutes of Health

Today the NIH includes 24 institutes, centers and divisions and has a $12 billion annual operating budget. More than half of the NIH extramural grants go to researchers at medical schools.

While NIH internal research has contributed significantly to medical science, it was the agency's extramural grant-making authority that transformed American medicine.

In 1944, President Franklin D. Roosevelt signed the Public Health Service Act, specifically giving the NIH authority to award grants for nonfederal research.

The American public was hungry for medical advancement. Already they'd seen what sulfa drugs and penicillin had done for soldiers wounded in war.

Soldiers "got very good medical care perhaps for the first time in their lives, and when they went home they didn't want to lose it," said Victoria Harden, historian at the NIH and an expert on the history of 20th century biomedical research.

The Only Way

At the same time, private philanthropic support of medical research had dropped off since the Great Depression, making government funds all the more necessary.

Also, with the public unwilling to support a national health insurance program, "there was no other way to improve American health at that moment" except by funding research that could lead to cures for infectious diseases, Harden said.

But it wasn't as easy as just pumping money into the research world.

"Science did not want government money," Harden said, noting that many researchers believed "anybody who lives on government money is bound to be corrupted. Government money was an anathema."

As a solution, a peer-review process by which expert panels judged the merits of research proposals was born. The process served as a buffer between Congress' appropriating powers and the research community.

"That's been the real genius of the NIH . . . [and] very much the reason we have accomplished as much as we have," Korn said.

"Competition [for research dollars] fosters creativity and raises the level of excellence," added Ralph Muller, president of the University of Chicago Hospitals.

Teaching Hospitals

With NIH grants available, it became expected that medical-school faculty would include trained scientists capable of doing biomedical research and therefore of winning NIH grants.

"The teaching hospitals got swept up into this new set of expectations" because the faculty conducting research were the same people treating hospital patients, Korn said.

Clinical programs, in turn, came to reflect the research done at the hospitals.

For example, University of Chicago researchers' immunology studies taught them about what leads a body to reject transplanted organs. Eventually, that knowledge enabled the university's hospital to have a leading liver transplant program, Muller said.

In his view, "It's the growth of the NIH funding that has led to advances in patient care."

Congress and President Clinton apparently agree. Clinton has proposed increasing the NIH budget 50 percent over five years. The Senate wants to double funding during the same period.

"Everybody wants the results," Muller said. "The public is demanding . . . that we cure these diseases."

"A PLACE FOR OURSELVES"

Black Hospitals Were the Pride of an Excluded Community

by Philip Dunn

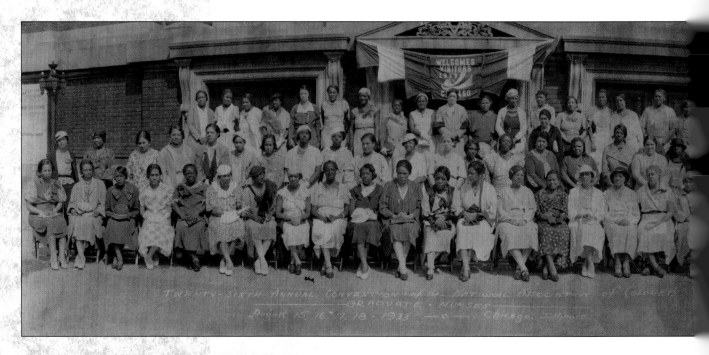

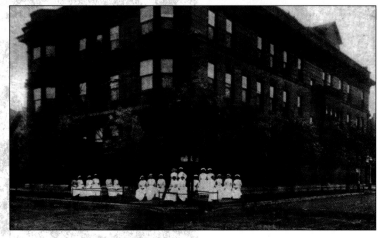

Women attending the 26th annual convention of the National Association of Colored Graduate Nurses in Chicago in August 1933 gathered for the above photo, which appeared in the Chicago Defender, *a black-owned newspaper.*

Left: Provident Hospital is shown in a vintage photo.

Source: Provident Hospital of Cook County

Many hospitals, from prestigious medical centers to tiny community clinics, at one time did not admit black patients and did not hire or train black doctors or nurses. Others confined black patients to "colored" wings. In the African-American community, those institutions are still sometimes known as "white" hospitals.

"In the minds of our grandparents, black and white, that's just the way it was," says Nathaniel Wesley Jr., assistant professor, Division of Health Care Management, School of Allied Health Services at Florida A&M University. "It was a way of life."

So, African-Americans built their own hospitals. Black-owned or -operated hospitals were prominent in the

South and in northern cities from the time of slavery until the Civil Rights era of the early 1960s.

"Originally created to provide health care and education within a segregated society, they evolved to become symbols of black pride and achievement," writes Vanessa Northington Gamble, M.D., author of *Making a Place for Ourselves: The Black Hospital Movement, 1920 to 1945.*

"They supplied medical care, provided training opportunities, and contributed to the development of a black professional class."

In the pre-Civil War South, a few large plantations assembled clinics for slaves. In 1832, in Savannah, GA, the first white-run hospital for blacks, the Georgia Infirmary, was established "for relief and protection of aged and afflicted Africans," Gamble writes.

After the war, whites built segregated hospitals for blacks. The movement changed radically in 1891 in Chicago, when Dr. Daniel Hale Williams, a black surgeon, established Provident Hospital and Training School on the city's South Side.

"Some members of the black community accused [Williams] of perpetuating segregation," Gamble writes. "One minister went so far as to curse the building and pray that it would burn to the ground. Williams was able to overcome such criticism because of the wide biracial support that the hospital received.

"Furthermore, the founder perceived the hospital not as an exclusively black enterprise, but as an interracial one that would not practice racial discrimination with regard to staff privileges, nurse training school applicants and the admission of patients."

Four years later, Williams helped found the National Medical Association (NMA), the nation's largest black doctors association. In 1908, black nurses—who also counted on black hospitals for training—formed the

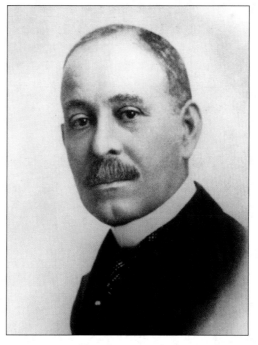

Daniel Hale Williams, a pioneer in heart surgery, founded Provident Hospital and Training School on Chicago's South Side in 1891.
Source: Corbis-Bettmann

National Association of Colored Graduate Nurses. The nurses group disbanded in 1951, apparently prematurely; 20 years later, the National Black Nurses Association was formed. Black hospitals flourished, their numbers hitting 118 in 1919, Gamble writes. In 1923, the NMA formed the National Hospital Association (NHA) to encourage establishment of black hospitals. In all, about 500 were established.

Like many older African-American doctors, St. Louis obstetrician and NMA President Nathaniel Murdoch, M.D., honed his skills at a black hospital. Murdoch trained at Homer G. Phillips Hospital in St. Louis, a city-owned, black-operated hospital that closed in 1979.

"This was a great training ground for black residents," he says.

The number of black hospitals fell rapidly when black physicians gained admitting privileges to white hospitals starting after World War II, and communities no longer felt the need to support such institutions. The National Hospital Association succumbed in the early 1940s when the NMA did not support it.

A few black hospitals remain. Scholars are left to argue over their legacy.

"They are proud symbols within the community," says Florida A&M's Wesley, former director of planning at Howard University Hospital, Washington, DC. "We can look at them and say, 'Yes, we have done this for ourselves.' "

To Murdoch, the decline of black hospitals bodes ill.

"We were never, in my opinion, amalgamated into American society," Murdoch says. "I think we should have things of our own, hospitals that are just as good as anybody else's hospital, residency programs as good as anybody's residency programs."

But others are not as concerned.

"They served a purpose, but as society changed, that purpose began to dwindle," says Elliott C. Roberts Sr., a Louisiana State University Medical Center professor and chairman of the Institute for Diversity in Health Management. "It's just like any other business. If you can't attract the customers, that says something."

PAGING DR. KILDARE

Today's Pop Culture Has Knocked Health Care Off Its Fictional Pedestal

by Jon Asplund

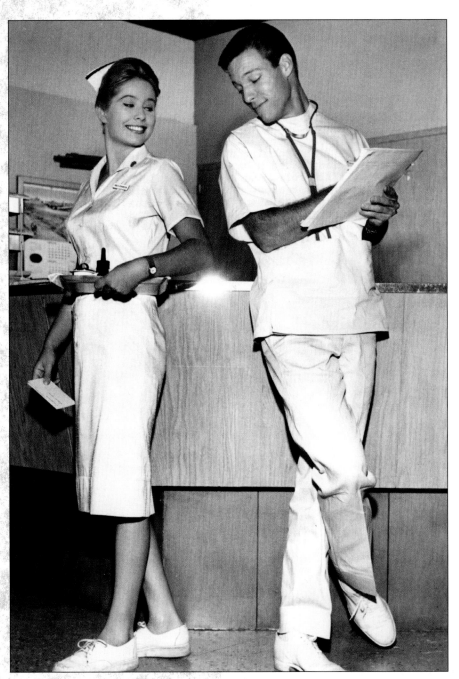

"@#% HMO *&#@$!" But the string of profanities Helen Hunt levels at HMOs isn't the most shocking health care reference in *As Good As It Gets*.

Viewers of the Oscar-nominated film are even more surprised to see a doctor making a house call in contemporary America.

Hunt plays a single mother whose son has chronic asthma. She blames her HMO for substandard treatment after a rich benefactor sends a big-shot specialist to take care of the boy.

But the HMO line has hit a nerve. Some managed care backers have described the scene as unrealistic, arguing that the best health plans know that quality preventive care saves money in the long run.

Many of those attending a recent health plan association meeting in Washington, DC, pointed to Hunt's invective as an example of "unfair" media bias.

The portrayal of health care in movies, television and novels has changed with the times. In general, the entertainment industry today presents a much more cynical view of medicine than it did in the past.

Critical Care, a black comedy released in 1997, offers biting commentary about the state of contemporary health care.

Actors James Spader and Albert Brooks are doctors at a hospital that hooks patients up to respirators, feeding tubes and every other gadget that will sustain life—as long as the patient has insurance.

But Brooks, as a department head emeritus, refuses to send his protege, Spader, to the emergency room to treat an uninsured patient.

Screenwriter and co-producer Steven Schwartz says the movie presents an "important discussion of what's the quality of life vs. the quantity of life."

While Schwartz stresses that he doesn't believe all doctors are nefarious enough to consider a patient's insurance before saving his or her life, or unnecessarily prolonging it, he does think the discussion of medicine has been skewed in the past.

"There's a long history of the doctor as Greek god," Schwartz says.

In 1954, "Janet Dean: Registered Nurse" told a young Sal Mineo not to worry about paying for his operation, that the hospital would pick up the tab.

In the television series, actress Ella Raines stood by doctors as they helped out poor kids or taught haughty New England socialites to respect "foreign" doctors.

Ten years later, that dreamboat Dr. Kildare, played by Richard Chamberlain, was TV's square-jawed, heroic physician at fictional Blair General Hospital.

"A thoroughly admirable physician, calm, objective, in control of himself, serving humanity with restraint and understanding," Kildare described himself, only somewhat sarcastically, after taking the law into his own hands to track down a fellow doctor's attacker.

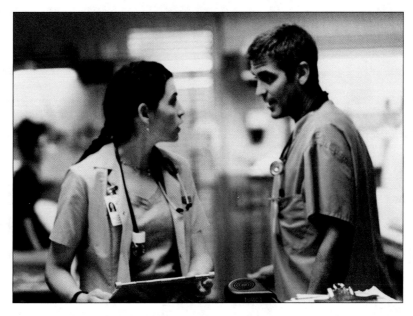

Getting serious. *In the 1950s, Dr. Kildare (facing page) took medicine far more lightly than does the 1990s' hospital drama* ER *(above). Then again, Dr. Kildare never signed a managed care contract.*

Sources: Corbis-Bettmann, facing page; Warner Brothers, above.

The episode does show the doctor with human frailties—by letting his emotions make him a heroic tough guy—and it includes a female physician, which was groundbreaking for that day and age.

It took a comedy in the 1970s to break the mold of the doctor as paragon of virtue and duty.

M*A*S*H dealt with more traumatic situations than perhaps any other hospital-based television show. But it did so with a healthy dose of gallows humor.

As doctors in a Korean War mobile army hospital, the characters were "irreverent, more human, raucous, disrespectful and fun," said Larry Gelbart, creator of the long-running comedy. "They took their work extremely seriously, but the rest of their lives was up for grabs. They weren't working on sick people, they were patching up soldiers to go back out on the battlefield. So they question the wastefulness of it and their role in it."

In the 1980s, the television program *St. Elsewhere* depended on its many characters' imperfections—from the trivial and to the very serious—for humor and drama.

One doctor had a habit of blowing up a latex glove over his head (and, Howie Mandel, the actor who played him, has gone on to a career in standup comedy). Another of the doctors turned out to be a serial rapist.

And today, we can watch an HIV-positive physician assistant work side by side with the—admittedly heroic—doctor who cannot stop smoking on *ER*, the NBC series that has climbed the ratings summit on the shoulders of its multifaceted characters.

DIPLOMA MILL DOCS

Landmark Flexner Report Finally Gives Fly-by-Night Medical Schools the Boot

by Matthew Weinstock

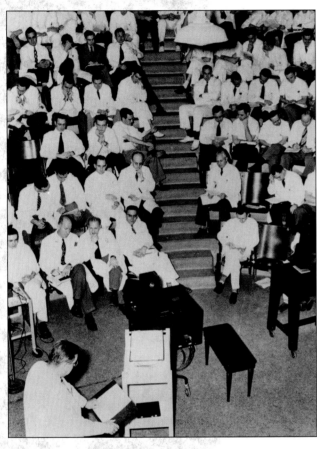

This photo, taken in 1949, shows Duke University physicians and medical students at a clinical pathological conference in which they reviewed findings from autopsies.

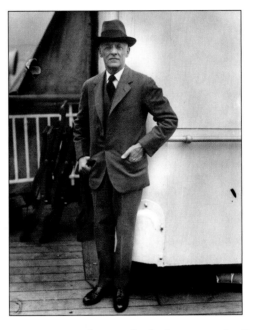

A 1910 report about medical education in the United States and Canada by noted educator Abraham Flexner (above) spurred a public outcry that resulted in higher standards for legitimate institutions and marked the beginning of the end for disreputable schools. The photo was taken upon Flexner's return to the United States in 1929 from a lecture tour of Europe. Historically, American medical students had spent most of their time in lecture halls, with little or no exposure to clinical settings. That changed dramatically after the reform movement took hold.

Source: Corbis-Bettmann

Guilt by association can be a powerful motivator. Such was the case in the late 1800s when the reputations of venerable medical schools were tarnished by schools of questionable quality.

Because medical education then was largely unregulated, there was great disparity among teaching institutions. At most medical schools, admission requirements were minimal, at best. Course work consisted of little more than a series of lectures and no actual clinical work.

"There was no contact with patients. Learning was all didactic," said Kenneth Ludmerer, M.D., professor of medicine in the School of Medicine at Washington University in St. Louis. Educators at elite schools saw that the entire profession was being hurt, he said.

After being appointed president of Harvard University in 1869, Charles W. Eliot said, "The whole system of medical education in this country needs thorough reformation."

He was more critical in his second annual report:

"It seems almost incredible that the grossly inadequate training should be the recognized preparation for aspirants to a profession that was once called learned, and which pre-eminently demands a mind well stored and a judgment well trained—a profession in which ignorance is criminality, and skill a benefaction—a profession which penetrates the most sacred retreats of human love, joy and sorrow, and deals daily with the issues of life and death."

Eliot's call for reforms met with limited success: Harvard and other elite institutions established a three-year progressive curriculum, extended courses from four months to a full year, and mandated smaller classes.

What really inspired reformers, though, was the establishment of the School of Medicine at Johns Hopkins University in 1893. The school set a new standard for medical education, wrote Vernon Lippard, M.D., dean emeritus of the Yale School of Medicine, in his book, *Half a Century of American Medical Education, 1920–1970.*

It was the first to hire full-time faculty. Previously, teachers were practicing physicians who were not dependent on the schools for their incomes and who showed little allegiance to the universities.

Johns Hopkins also established its own hospital and introduced clinical clerkships. And students had contact with patients, not just books.

Still, change was incremental and medical education had yet to earn the public's confidence. In fact, it often was ridiculed.

In 1909, Mark Twain, upon being awarded an honorary medical degree by the New York Postgraduate Medical School, remarked, "I am glad to be among my own kind tonight. I was once a sharpshooter, but now I practice a much higher and equally as deadly a profession."

Reformers needed a national movement to weed out the bad apples and inspire public confidence, according to Ludmerer.

That came courtesy of the Carnegie Foundation for the Advancement of Teaching, which was asked by the American Medical Association (AMA) to assess the state of medical education in North America.

The foundation selected Abraham Flexner, an expert on education systems, as its chief inspector. After a crash course on medical education with help from colleagues at Johns Hopkins and the AMA, he set off to visit all 155 medical schools in the United States and Canada.

He found a system in disarray. The lack of standards, mostly didactic teaching methods and limited resources had a dramatic impact on the quality of graduates.

"[T]here is probably no other country in the world in which there is so great a distance and so fatal a difference between the best, the average, and the worst," he wrote in his 1910 report, *Medical Education in the United States and Canada.*

Flexner's report incited public outrage.

"All the honest schools wanted to teach medicine the way Flexner suggested and many were," Ludmerer said. "Flexner helped arouse public support and money to build up quality education programs."

Money from private foundations started to pour into elite institutions. Average schools adopted Flexner's ideas. Admission requirements were strengthened and teaching moved from lecture halls to clinical settings. Throughout the next decade, most fly-by-night schools closed their doors.

"There is a great myth that there was nothing but darkness before Flexner. That is false," Ludmerer said. "What Flexner did was bring a lot of these reform issues to the public. He made it a public rather than professional issue, and that helped push things."

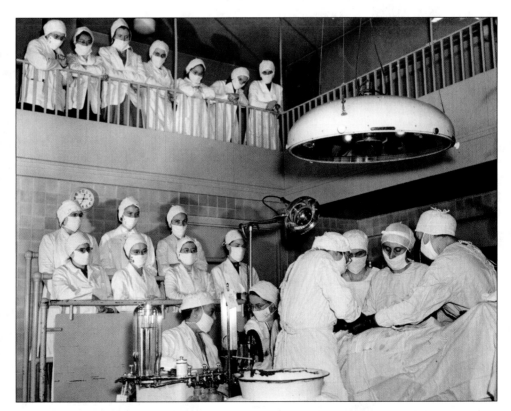

Students at the Women's Medical College in Philadelphia watch a surgeon perform an operation in 1946. Source: Corbis-Bettmann

PARENT COMPANY

From Malted Milk to Insurance, Ward's Watched Out for Employees' Health

by Jack Bess

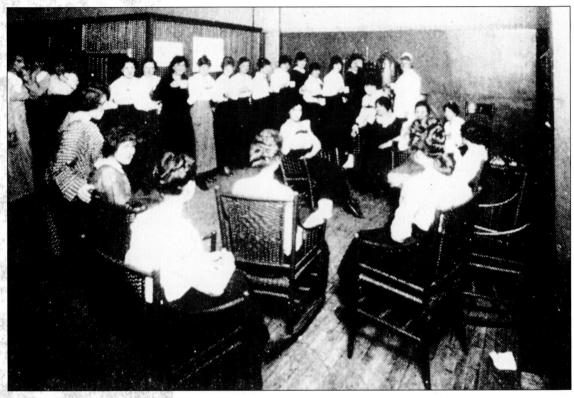

During the Depression, Montgomery Ward provided malted-milk breaks for employees, many of whom needed the energy boost because they weren't getting enough to eat at home.   Source: Montgomery Ward Archives

The Chicago company that revolutionized retailing with the mail-order catalog also pioneered a form of insurance for its employees that became the blueprint for group health plans.

On July 1, 1912, an innovation called the group insurance policy was issued to 2,912 employees of Montgomery Ward & Co. by the Equitable Life Assurance Society of the United States. Ward's bought $5,946,564 in life insurance coverage for employees who had worked with the company for five or more years. Written as a life insurance plan, Ward's policy included health and disability benefits.

News of the insurance contract hit the front page of the *New York Times* almost three months earlier, on April 13. The newspaper reported that this new "blanket policy

under what is known as the group plan" was the largest policy ever written in the United States.

In a follow-up story the next day, the *Times* reported that Ward's policy had sparked "considerable discussion" among large companies intrigued by the economies of group insurance, which included dispensing with individual medical exams, solicitation and fee collecting.

The *Times* reported, "This wide divergence from ordinary insurance methods is based on the theory that a group is acceptable as a whole, the company can take the risk of any members of the group not up to the rigid medical standard required in individual cases."

Ironically, even though Ward's is credited with the first group insurance plan, when it came to implementing the policy, the company actually was beaten to the punch by an Equitable official apparently inspired by Wards' concept.

Special Care for Employees

Providing insurance was just one way that Ward proved to be a conscientious employer, according to a corporate history, *A Century of Serving Customers, 1872–1972: The Story of Montgomery Ward*, by Frank Latham.

The company had medical staffs in its offices, including three doctors and four nurses in its Chicago plant, and a dental department to serve its employees.

Latham provides other examples of the company's paternalism: On rainy days, when female employees arrived for work in soaking clothes, the company provided them with stockings and skirts to wear while their own clothes were drying. Women were allowed to leave work earlier than the men so they could get seats on the street-car. Ward's also had an educational division that held evening classes for its workers in English (for recent immigrants) and business subjects.

And, Latham wrote, "Because pulmonary tuberculosis was a serious problem in those days, girls who had colds and were under-weight were served 12-ounce glasses of malted milk at 10 a.m. and 3 p.m. Men and boys with similar ailments were also served."

Even before Ward's group plan was created, employees had access to some illness and death benefits. Starting in 1894, an association called the Clerks Benefit Society paid claims drawing on monthly dues paid by several hundred Ward's workers. Additional funds would be raised at company dances.

Group Policies Catch On

After the turn of the century, Charles Thorne, son of company co-founder Robert Thorne, began talking to insurance companies about a new kind of

Under the leadership of President Charles H. Thorne (top), Montgomery Ward became the first major company to provide group life insurance for its employees. The policy (right) was issued on July 1, 1912, by the Equitable Life Assurance Society.

Source: Montgomery Ward Archives

life insurance policy that would cover treatment for sickness, accidents and old age. All rejected the proposal, until Equitable decided to consider it. But by early 1911, the initiative had stalled.

According to Latham, one of Equitable's directors was sold on the idea of group coverage and decided to adopt it for his Pantasole Leather Company in Passaic (NJ), which employed 121 people. This development prompted a new Equitable official to reopen talks with Thorne, and paved the way for Ward's own contract.

Disability and pension coverage were separated and handled by the London Guarantee and Accident Company. Employees contributed 3 percent of their weekly wages, which covered half of the policy's total cost.

"The plan paid for funeral expenses, a year's wages to the beneficiary of an unmarried employee and annuities of 25 percent of the wages to the widow of an employee, plus 20 to 25 percent for her minor child or children," Latham wrote.

Equitable President W.A. Day promoted group insurance as a means to expand coverage to those who might be risky to insure individually. The "general character of the group" must be investigated, as individuals would be examined if they were to be insured separately.

"Between the individually insurable and the individually noninsurable, between the young, the middle-aged and the old, the employer draws no distinction," Day said, "and any scheme that would completely cover employees must take them all, the young with the old, the weak with the strong, depending upon the underlying averages that make insurance possible and supply its reasons for existence."

Disability coverage lasted only until 1941, when the London casualty company discontinued the policy. In its place, Ward's sponsored the Employee's Mutual Benefit Society that, like the earlier clerk's association, paid claims with monthly dues.

HAUNTED BY POLIO

Decades Later, Many Survivors Relive Devastating Symptoms

by Betty A. Marton

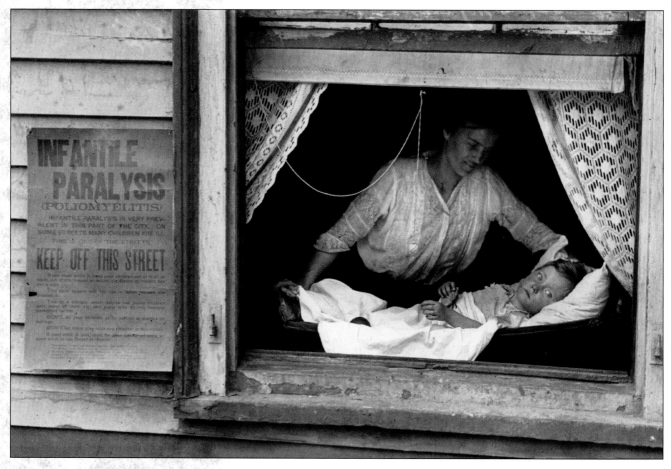

Quarantined by order of the local health department, a child stricken by polio can view the world only through a parlor window while his mother stands by sadly. A health department sign nailed to the outside of their home warns passersby to keep away. This photo was taken in the summer of 1916. Source: Corbis-Bettmann

The afternoon she returned home after voting for Adlai Stevenson in 1952, Ruth Stein knew she was sick. Within days, the weakness she had been feeling turned to paralysis and the 29-year-old mother of two was unable to move from the waist down.

Her doctor took her to New York City's Lenox Hill Hospital where a spinal tap revealed that she had contracted polio.

"It was the last big year of polio," Stein recalled, "but because I was an adult, they had a hard time figuring out what it was."

Stein stayed at Lenox Hill in a iron-barred, broom-closet-sized room where few people, including nurses, dared come near her to try to help relieve her excruciating pain. She returned home shortly before Christmas with leg braces, a wheelchair, crutches and "great, big horrible shoes" that frightened her 3-year-old daughter.

Stein was one of the lucky ones. Through the Polio Foundation, she worked twice a day with a physiotherapist, a former ballet dancer from Russia, and a year and a half later, she was able to walk independently.

The virus that befell Stein has caused paralysis and death for much of human history. References to polio first appeared in a 3,000-year-old Egyptian stone engraving and extend through the 1950s, when vaccines developed by Jonas Salk, M.D., and Albert Sabin, M.D., rapidly eradicated the disease throughout most of the industrialized world.

Polio, which attacks the central nervous system, is easily transmitted by infected raw sewage in public water supplies. Ironically, the outbreaks that plagued this country in the first half of the century correlated with improved sanitation and living conditions.

Before indoor plumbing, virtually all infants were exposed to the virus, when the infection was most likely to be asymptomatic and confer lifelong immunity to the disease. Older children or adults who were infected were more likely to be paralyzed or killed by the virus.

Until President Franklin D. Roosevelt, who had polio, declared a war on the virus, it was considered an "immigrants' disease."

The children who were its primary victims were feared by society, isolated from their parents and helped, if at all, only by private charitable organizations.

Paying for the Past

Now, nearly half a century since this part of the world experienced its last polio epidemic, approximately 60 percent of the 640,000 survivors are suffering once again from the disease they thought they had put behind them decades ago.

"Many polio survivors are having significantly disabling health problems, such as weakness, fatigue, pain and declining functional abilities that seem to stem from

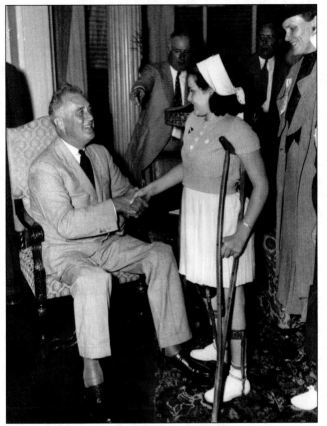

President Franklin D. Roosevelt greets polio survivor Betty June Berger of Rosiclare, IL, in September 1936. Until FDR, himself paralyzed by polio, declared war on the virus, many Americans considered it a disease of immigrants.

Source: Corbis-Bettmann

degenerating polio damaged nerves and muscles," said Frederick M. Maynard, M.D., head of physical medicine rehabilitation at Case Western Reserve University Medical School/ Metro Health, Cleveland.

Diagnosing post-polio syndrome is largely a process of exclusion because there is no test, Maynard said. Its symptoms are often intertwined with other age-related problems, making it difficult to define.

The lack of knowledge and understanding about the syndrome compounds patients' misery, said Sheila Lujen, who heads a foundation for post-polio patients.

"Most doctors today are unaware of [post-polio syndrome] and don't know what to do with us," said Lujen, who contracted a rare case of polio after swimming in a polluted lagoon in 1968 when she was 13. "Most of the older physicians who diagnosed and treated polio have passed on and obtaining older medical records is next to impossible."

Now in her late 70s, Ruth Stein still works full time, and says her health complaints are no worse than those of most people her age.

Lujen continues to suffer from scoliosis and now experiences weakness in her hands and arms, loss of balance, and swallowing and breathing difficulties. She is determined to shed light on the phenomenon that Maynard says is documented in 19th century literature but still largely unrecognized by today's medical community.

"We have made a lot of progress recognizing post-polio syndrome in the last 10 years and realizing that it doesn't always respond to therapies the way other diseases do with the same symptoms," Maynard said, "but the medical community does not yet see it as a true, new disease."

HE HAD A BIG HEART

*Barney Clark's Physical Weakness Made His Artificial Heart
Necessary, but His Psychological Strength Made Him a Hero*

by Betty A. Marton

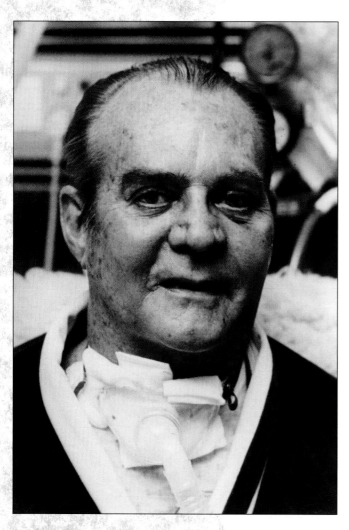

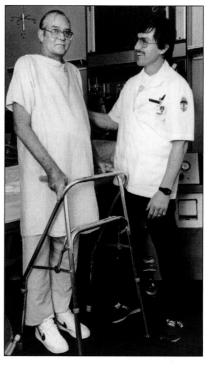

*Two months after the operation, Clark was strong enough to
navigate the intensive care unit using a walker. However, he
suffered a series of setbacks and required three additional operations. He died on March 23, 1983, his artificial heart still
beating in his chest. Clark was eulogized as a "seemingly ordinary man who became a selfless pioneer."*

Source: J. Willard Marriott Library, University of Utah. Photographs
by Brad Nelson.

During the 112 days he lived tethered by 6-foot
hoses to the air compressor that powered his artificial heart, Barney Clark made medical history.
Without the polyurethane and aluminum Jarvik-7 heart
implanted in the 62-year-old retired dentist, he would
have died in December 1982.

From the outset, Clark embarked upon the experiment
less for the time it might buy him than the contribution
he could make to medical science.

"I don't think he really felt it would succeed," said his
son, Stephen K. Clark, M.D. "His interest in going ahead

was to make this contribution. Helping others was one of
his strong motivations."

Clark took it upon himself to understand the implications of being implanted with the device invented by
Robert Jarvik, M.D. He was described by the University
of Utah Medical Center's selection committee as a
"bright, articulate, knowledgeable candidate who under-
stands the importance of the operation and who wants to
make a contribution to medical science."

He observed the implantation of the Jarvik-7 heart in
an animal and entered the ordeal prepared for any

outcome. Realizing that he would die if the operation was not successful, he put his affairs in order.

His wife, Una Loy, hoped the operation would succeed enough that he would one day leave the hospital. So she moved from Seattle to a house in Salt Lake City designed to accommodate the 375-pound compressor that powered her husband's new heart.

A Grueling Ordeal

On the brink of death, his own dying heart unable to pump enough blood and paper-thin from earlier steroid therapy, Clark signed two federally mandated consent forms 24 hours apart.

The seven-and-a-half-hour operation began early on the morning of Dec. 2, 1982. Surgeons, led by William C. DeVries, M.D., removed about two-thirds of Clark's diseased heart. They extracted the left and right ventricles—the bottom two chambers—and anchored the artificial heart to the upper left and right atria.

The artificial heart made a soft clicking sound audible through Clark's chest wall. It was adjusted frequently during the first days.

By February, Clark was able to use a walker and pedal an exercise bicycle for up to 10 minutes, but he was never able to leave the hospital. Within days of the operation he suffered one setback after another, including seizures and aspiration pneumonia complicated by emphysema, and kidney and pulmonary failure.

He required three additional operations: to stop air leaks from his lungs, replace a broken part of the artificial

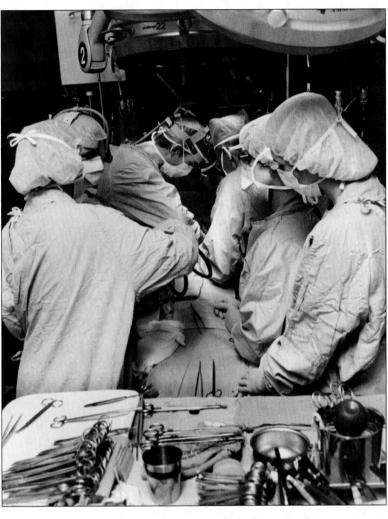

Early in the morning of Dec. 2, 1982, a team of physicians and nurses at the University of Utah Medical Center begin a 7 1/2-hour operation to implant the Jarvik-7 artificial heart into Barney Clark.

Source: J. Willard Marriott Library, University of Utah. Photograph by Brad Nelson.

heart and stop a severe nosebleed. Clark often depended on a mechanical respirator to breathe deeply. When not connected to the respirator, he was able to speak only by covering the tracheotomy tube in his windpipe.

With the eyes of the world on him, Clark had submitted to a life of complete vulnerability, dependency and uncertainty, which, despite his enormous psychological strength, as well as the unflinching support of his wife and children, resulted in "intensive care unit psychosis."

For some weeks after the operation, he withdrew from those responsible for his care, making only infrequent eye contact with others. Chase N. Petersen, M.D., vice president of health affairs at the University of Utah, tried to illustrate how a patient might be affected by the circumstances Clark endured.

"Stand up here, let us take off your clothes, make you unable to speak very well, put needles and tubes into you, have night indistinguishable from day over a several-week period, and then I'll ask if by any chance you are frustrated and confused," he said.

Clark's artificial heart was still working when he died from circulatory collapse and multiple organ failure on March 23, 1983.

He was eulogized as "a seemingly ordinary man who became a selfless pioneer," by John Dwan, spokesman for the University of Utah Medical Center. "He did a service to mankind and the knowledge that we will gain from him will serve us all," Dwan said.

STEADY BURN

First Inspection Reports Went Up in Flames,
but Hospitals Still Feel the Heat

by Susan Powers

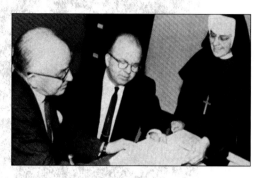
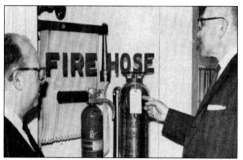
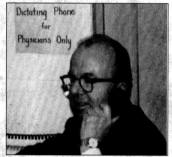
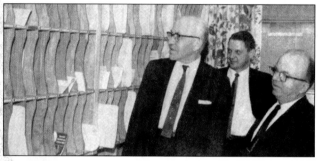
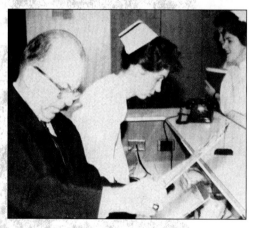

In 1961, both health care and inspections by the Joint Commission on Accreditation of Hospitals (JCAH) were far less sophisticated than they are today. These photographs, which appeared in the March 1961 issue of Hospital Management, show a new JCAH surveyor, Arno Fromm, M.D., on a training survey at Oak Park (IL) Hospital. Clockwise from top left: Sister St. Marcienne, the hospital administrator, presents minutes of the governing board to Denver Vickers, M.D., JCAH assistant director, and Fromm; Fromm and Vickers check the inspection date on a fire extinguisher; Jack Tope, M.D., center, points out that despite a shortage of interns only a few medical charts are unfinished thanks to modern dictating equipment installed the previous year; and in the final two photos, Fromm inspects medical records and dictating equipment.

Source: AHA archive

The first standard was little more than a piece of paper stating that hospitals should keep good records. And the results of the first hospital surveys were so poor that they were destroyed.

Today, the Accreditation Manual for Hospitals is 4 inches thick and contains more than 500 standards. And hospital survey results are published on the Internet for everyone to read.

While a lot of things have changed at the Joint Commission on Accreditation of Healthcare Organizations (JCAHO), the goal has been the same since 1910, when Ernest Codman, M.D., proposed a system that would track every hospital patient to determine standardized treatment protocol.

The Joint Commission was created at a time when there was nothing to help hospitals and physicians systematically assess and improve the quality of service and care, said Tom Granatir, director of the AHA's quality initiatives.

JCAHO was formally founded in 1951, but it dates to Codman's 1910 proposal which helped launch the

American College of Surgeons (ACS) in 1913. The ACS used Codman's end-result system of hospitalization proposal as its stated objective.

By 1917, the ACS had developed the "Minimum Standard for Hospitals"—a one-page list of requirements—and began on-site inspections. Results from the first year of inspections were horrifying; only 89 out of 692 hospitals met the requirements. The results were so bad that the group of surgeons reviewing the results took them to the basement of New York City's Waldorf Hotel where they were meeting and burned them in the furnace.

"They didn't want to sink the birthing of a program of accreditation standards to improve patient care," said William Kridelbaugh, M.D., past chairman of the ACS board of commissioners.

Over the next 10 years, the ACS compiled and printed the first standards manual consisting of 18 pages; by 1950, 3,200 hospitals had met the standards outlined under the program.

That same year, the ACS announced that it could no longer afford to administer the program and requested that the AHA take over.

"I knew one thing," recalled George Bugbee, then AHA executive director. If the program was to continue, "hospitals better jump in and be in favor of it and keep it alive," Bugbee said, in Lewis E. Weeks' hospital administration oral history series sponsored by the AHA.

The Joint Commission Is Born

A year of meetings between doctors and hospitals resulted in the creation of the Joint Commission on Accreditation of Hospitals—an independent, not-for-profit organization formed to provide voluntary hospital accreditation. Representatives included the AHA, the ACS, the American College of Physicians, the American Medical Association and the Canadian Medical Association, which later withdrew to form a similar national group.

This new commission published its *Standards for Hospital Accreditation* and began accrediting hospitals in January 1953.

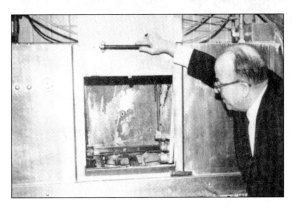

Fromm inspects an oven (top) and dishwasher (bottom).

Source: AHA archive

In 1965, Congress fueled the commission's growth by passing the Medicare Act. The act included a provision stating that hospitals accredited by the Joint Commission would be "deemed" to be in compliance with most of the Medicare Conditions of Participation for Hospitals, allowing them to participate in Medicare and Medicaid.

By the mid-1970s, the commission had expanded accreditation to include long-term care, psychiatric facilities, substance-abuse programs, community mental-health programs and ambulatory care.

In 1987, the commission's name was changed to the Joint Commission on Accreditation of Healthcare Organizations to reflect the expanding health care delivery system.

While the philosophy of accreditation had transformed from "a minimum standard of care" to "optimal achievable levels of quality," the JCAHO's most dramatic philosophical changes occurred in 1986.

"People wanted quantitative information on health care organizations and physicians," said Dennis O'Leary, M.D., executive director of the commission. JCAHO responded with its "Agenda for Change."

The agenda addressed concerns about the effect of cost-cutting on quality of care. It did so retooling the objectives of accreditation, the criteria for evaluation, the operational process, public disclosure and the use of performance measurement. "We didn't merely tweak the old process," O'Leary said. "We started with a blank sheet of paper and redid the process."

Amid growing interest in quality, JCAHO recently implemented a so-called ORYX policy that requires health care organizations to report outcomes measurements and a sentinel-events initiative to create a database about serious accidents in the health care setting.

Today, JCAHO evaluates and accredits more than 18,000 U.S. health care organizations and programs. It employs more than 500 medical professionals to conduct the surveys and another 500 to administer programs. It is governed by a 28-member board of commissioners.

For the Public Good

With Prodding, Congress Finally Regulated the Food and Drug Industries in 1906

by Jack Bess

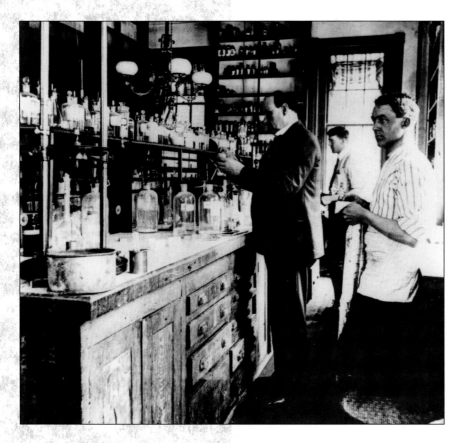

Harvey Washington Wiley, a dogged campaigner for federal regulation of the food and drug industries since becoming chief chemist of the U.S. Department of Agriculture in 1883, visited one of the government laboratories where in 1902 he tested the effects of then-unregulated food preservatives such as borax, formaldehyde and saltpeter on robust, young volunteers. The press dubbed Wiley and his team the poison squad.

Source: Corbis-Bettmann

Government can react quickly in the heat of crisis or slowly enough to span decades. Illustrations of each mode can be found in the origins of the U.S. Centers for Disease Control and Prevention (CDC) and of the Food and Drug Administration (FDA). The CDC grew out of a World War II-era program to control malaria, and the agency still functions as a rapid-response operation.

By contrast, it took several decades for Congress to recognize the need for a national pure-food and drug law. More than 100 such bills died in Congress until the first food and drug legislation was passed in 1906, and the FDA's precursor was formed to enforce it.

What helped set the stage for the 1906 law was an experiment that, in retrospect, sounds like a "Geraldo"-style stunt.

Its formal name was the "hygienic table," but newspapers referred to the 1902 effort led by U.S. government chemist Harvey Washington Wiley as the "poison squad."

Wiley had battled for pure-food legislation since becoming chief of the U.S. Department of Agriculture's Bureau of Chemistry in 1883. The nature of America's food supply had changed in the late 19th century because of leaps in industrialization and growing urban populations, Wiley wrote in his 1930 autobiography.

Preserved and canned foods were in demand. Sulphate of copper was added to canned vegetables to brighten their color, and sulphur dioxide was used in the bleaching of sugar.

Patent medicine was completely unregulated. Liver and gallstone "remedies" and the like were simply alcoholic drinks that made the customer crave more. Formulas advertised as pain-relief elixirs used narcotics, Wiley wrote, and "mothers doped their babies into insensibility at night with soothing syrups containing opium or morphine."

Individual states had passed food laws but there was no uniform national standard regulating the use of chemical preservatives and food coloring. Food canners and other commercial interests feared that such regulation would ruin their businesses.

With business interests arrayed against federal regulation, Congress shot down more than 100 pure-food and drug bills from 1879 to 1906.

Wiley had lectured, written and pushed for a national pure-food law, and in 1902 launched the experiment that seized national attention, and earned him praise but also ridicule on the vaudeville stage and in the press, where it was routinely referred to as the poison squad.

A special act in Congress allowed Wiley to assemble a group of 12 young men. These volunteers pledged to eat, for one year, only meals prepared in a small kitchen at the bureau headquarters. Their meals contained measured amounts of commonly used preservatives, including borax, formaldehyde and saltpeter. When a volunteer's digestion or health was impaired, Wiley gave him several days off to recuperate.

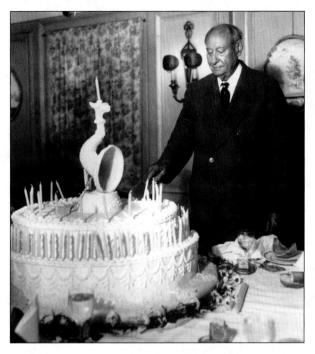

In 1926, at the age of 82, Wiley cuts a cake celebrating the federal Pure Food Laws, which Congress had passed 20 years prior. The industrialization and population shift of the late 1800s brought about a change in America's food supply, adding chemicals both to preserve certain food and to make it look fresher and more appealing. The federal Bureau of Chemistry initially was charged with enforcing the Pure Food Laws, but in 1927, the responsibility shifted to the newly created Food, Drug and Insecticide Administration, which became the Food and Drug Administration in 1931. Source: Corbis-Bettmann

Wiley reasoned that if "young, robust" volunteers suffered from the effects of adulterated food, "the deduction would naturally follow that children and older persons, more susceptible than they, would be greater sufferers from similar causes."

The law passed by Congress in 1906 defined "adulterated" and "misbranded" food and drugs, and prohibited their shipment across state lines. The Bureau of Chemistry was charged with enforcing it.

The bureau fought hundreds of court cases that established legal procedures and inspection techniques. In 1927, this responsibility was taken over by the newly created Food, Drug and Insecticide Administration, which became the FDA in 1931.

Still, food adulteration and patent-medicine remained a problem. In the 1930s, for instance, more than 100 people died from a conconction called "Elixir of Sulfanilamide."

In 1933, the New Deal administration sought to toughen the 1906 law. Industry and advertising opposition was so strong that it took members of congress five years to

craft and pass a new bill, the Federal Food, Drug, and Cosmetic Act of 1938.

Among other provisions, the law extended government regulation to cosmetics and therapeutic devices, and required drug companies to provide scientific proof that new drugs are safe before they are marketed. The FDA's workload grew when World War II spurred the development of new drugs such as antibiotics, which required testing by the agency.

War in Europe also prompted a government initiative that led to the formation of the CDC. In 1940, at the request of the War Department, the Public Health Service began a program to eradicate malaria around military camps in the U.S. South.

The fledgling Atlanta-based program, Malaria Control in War Areas (MCWA), employed not just physicians but engineers and entomologists. MCWA field workers dug ditches to drain swamps and sprayed areas with various larvicides such as the insecticide Paris Green, diesel oil and, in 1944, DDT.

During the war years, MCWA was deployed in 21 states, the District of Columbia and the Caribbean, and its mission expanded to tackle yellow fever, dengue and typhus.

Joseph Mountin, M.D., a Public Health Service official, successfully pushed for MCWA to have a role in postwar government. Launched in 1946 as the Communicable Disease Center, the agency continued its malaria work but gradually expanded its scope to cover such health problems as polio, venereal disease, smallpox and tuberculosis.

The current Centers for Disease Control and Prevention keeps vigil on emerging diseases around the globe. The agency's surveillance section, for example, strives to predict what form of virus will emerge in the coming flu season, while the CDC's Center for Infectious Diseases dispatches epidemiologists when such new or unusual illnesses as hantavirus and Legionnaires' disease appear.

LIVING LEGACIES

Not-So-Mad Scientists Took Organ Transplants from Frankenstein Fantasies to Routine Medicine

by Kevin Murray

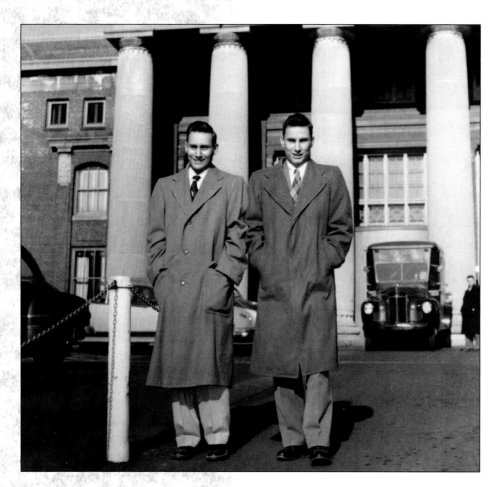

Twin brothers Richard and Ronald Herrick leave Peter Bent Brigham Hospital, Boston, Jan. 29, 1955, after their history-making kidney transplant. Ronald donated his kidney to Richard, who was suffering from nephritis.

Source: Corbis-Bettmann

Before the breakthroughs in surgical techniques and medications, organ transplantation in the United States was considered at best experimental, something seen mostly on late-night horror movies.

Pioneering efforts began in the late 1940s, with Australian scientist Sir Macfarlane Burnet, M.D., and British scientist Peter B. Medawar leading the way. Burnet and Medawar won the 1960 Nobel Prize in physiology and medicine for their efforts in transplant immunology.

The first successful kidney transplant was performed on identical twins at Boston's Peter Bent Brigham Hospital in 1954. Five years later, doctors there performed the first successful kidney transplant between nonidentical twins.

"Many transplant centers have patients who received transplanted kidneys in the 1950s who still have their kidneys today," said Bertram Kasiske, M.D., professor of medicine at the University of Minnesota.

In 1967, a human heart was transplanted at Groote Schuur Hospital in South Africa.

As techniques have evolved, transplants of every kind have become safer.

"However, the thing that has changed organ donation from an experimental to a routine procedure has been the dramatic improvement in immunosuppressive drugs that are used to help patients fight off rejection," Kasiske said.

The survival rates today are very good for all major types of organ transplantation. They continue to increase dramatically in kidney, heart and liver, the three most commonly transplanted organs. In 1996, physicians in the United States performed 11,099 kidney transplants, 4,058 liver transplants and 2,342 heart transplants, according to the United Network for Organ Sharing (UNOS).

Setting Up a Network
Under the National Organ Transplantation Act of 1984, Richmond, VA-based UNOS contracted with the federal Department of Health and Human Services (HHS) to establish and maintain a national organ procurement and transplantation network.

The move to coordinate nationally was a significant step in the evolution of organ transplantation, UNOS spokesman Joel Newman said.

"If we have a well-matched kidney out in New York and a patient in California, it is possible under a national registry system to have the kidney flown from New York to California," Newman said.

More lung and pancreas transplants are being performed, and those survival rates have increased significantly over the last few years.

Unfortunately, the supply of donors hasn't kept pace with the rapidly increasing need for organs.

"When [UNOS] started the organ-allocation contract with HHS, the waiting list for organs was 13,000," Newman said. "Today, 11 years later, the waiting list approaches 59,000."

In some years, "the waiting list would grow between 5 and 10 percent and the number of donors would grow between 1 and 5 percent," Newman said. "So, if you chart that out over time, the gap between donors and candidates grows wider and wider."

Informing the Public
Numerous public awareness campaigns have attempted to increase the supply of available organs. Those campaigns range from efforts at neighborhood churches to national television commercials featuring basketball superstar Michael Jordan.

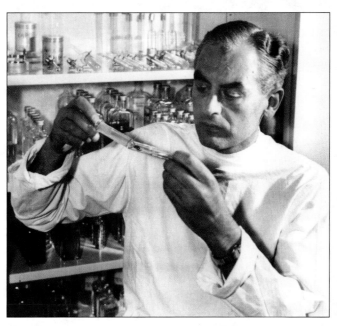

Peter B. Medawar works in his London laboratory in October 1960. Medawar and Australian Macfarlane Burnet, M.D., won the 1960 Nobel Prize in physiology and medicine for their efforts on transplant immunology. Source: Corbis-Bettmann

The efforts to educate people about what organ donation is all about, encouraging them to sign organ donation cards and informing family members—either verbally or through a living will—of their wishes to be an organ donor.

"The vast majority of adults in the U.S. never publicly signify their wishes—either positively or negatively—regarding organ donation," Newman said. "So, if there is no public declaration, the family often is left making a very difficult decision at the time of their loved one's death."

Newman said there is no magic bullet to cure the growing organ-shortage problem.

"Many people in the field believe this pool of potential donors is shrinking because of such factors as public-safety laws—mandatory seat-belt and helmet usage—and better trauma care and stroke medicine treatment," Newman said.

Organ-allocation policies are based on such factors as medical urgency, waiting times, and candidates who are biologically disadvantaged—rare blood type, growth or developmental problems, etc.—with such medical utility measures as ensuring high survival rates.

As organ transplants have evolved out of the realm of experimental procedures, the federal government and more insurance companies have agreed to cover the procedure.

"It is now routine for kidneys, and [it] has become more and more routine for other organs," Kasiske said.

However, there still are major issues regarding coverage, he said. For example, Medicare only covers immunosuppression medication for three years, but patients need to be able to take the drugs for the rest of their lives.

"A lot of people in this field believe there are patients who lose their transplants because they can't afford to take their medication," Kasiske said. "It always is hard to prove because most patients don't tell you that they're not taking their medication."

POPULAR MECHANICS

Nearly 50 Years Ago, a Frustrated Surgeon Built a Machine
That Changed Heart Surgery Forever

by Chris Larson

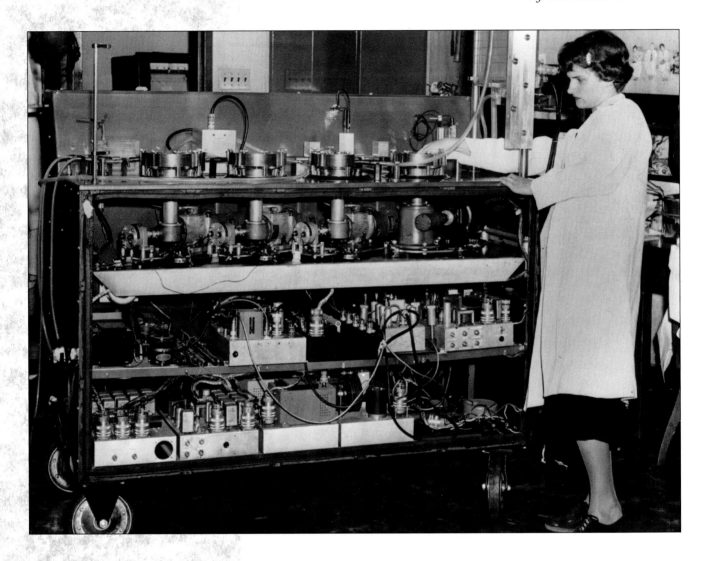

Surgery of the heart has probably reached the limits set by nature to all surgery: no new method and no new discovery can overcome the natural difficulties that attend a wound of the heart.

— Stephen Paget, *The Surgery of the Chest*, 1898

Paget's declaration reflected the view of the medical establishment at the end of the 19th century, but 100 years later, heart surgery is common. It's come so far because of a remarkable series of innovations and

new technologies that physicians of Paget's time could not have foreseen.

In the first decades of the 20th century, surgeons were operating on arteries and the lining around the heart. But with a few exceptions, the heart itself remained off-limits. Surgeons could expose the heart, but not without a tremendous loss of blood; even then, performing delicate maneuvers on a beating heart was extremely difficult. The heart could be stopped, but only for a few minutes or the patients suffered brain damage or died.

The situation began to change in the 1930s. Surgeons like John Gibbon, M.D., were frustrated by their inability to help patients with heart problems.

"Gibbon had a patient who died from a blood clot in her lungs," said Thoralf Sundt, M.D., a surgeon and associate professor at the Washington University School of Medicine, St. Louis. "Gibbon said, 'There's got to be a way that we can fix this problem.' It inspired him to find a solution."

The solution was in the nature of the heart itself. Because pumping blood is a mechanical process, surgeons wondered, why not temporarily replace the circulation with other mechanical devices, then stop the heart and operate on it?

Gibbon began developing machines that pumped blood from the heart and lungs into a chamber that added oxygen to the blood. Despite primitive working conditions—he bought pumps at secondhand stores, and snared stray cats in alleys for test subjects—his early heart-lung machines allowed cats to survive up to four hours with a stopped heart.

Gibbon's biggest problem was getting oxygen into the blood without damaging the blood cells, so his colleagues tried less mechanical methods. Surgeons had limited success with partial bypass—pumping blood around the heart but through the patient's lungs—in the early 1950s. Other researchers tried cross-circulation, moving the patient's blood through a healthy donor's heart and lungs. Still other trials involved a heart pump and a dog's or monkey's lung.

But Gibbon's machine ultimately proved the most effective. In May 1953—after nearly 20 years of research and refinements, just half a century after Paget said it couldn't be done—Gibbon performed the first successful heart surgery on a human with a heart-lung machine.

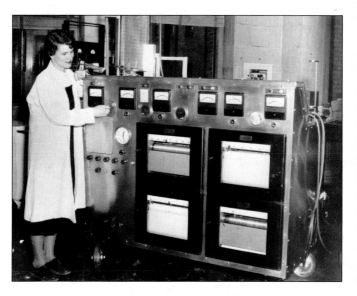

Clunky, but it worked. *It might not be slick by today's standards, but this heart-lung machine (shown above and on the facing page) invented by John H. Gibbon Jr., M.D., was the foundation of modern heart surgery. The apparatus was first used in May 1953 at Jefferson Medical College, Philadelphia, to pump and oxygenate the blood of an 18-year-old patient while surgeons sewed up the inner walls of her heart. Gibbon had begun to develop the machine 19 years earlier, buying parts at secondhand stores and using stray alley cats as test subjects.*

Source: Corbis-Bettmann

The machine wasn't perfect. It was bulky and complicated, and still damaged the blood. But it allowed surgery inside the heart. Later, surgeons made improvements, and the machine became widely used, particularly after 1965, when coronary bypass surgery was introduced.

"The heart-lung machine is the foundation of our specialty," Sundt said. "Heart surgery couldn't have grown the way it has without it."

Today's heart-lung machine still has drawbacks; damaged blood, clotting problems, lung damage and, occasionally, strokes. It's also expensive. All of which has inspired a search for alternatives. One of the most promising new developments is the stabilizer.

The stabilizer is remarkably simple: stainless steel and plastic instruments apply gentle pressure or suction to keep a small section of the heart—about 1 inch by 2 inches—from moving. Surgeons perform bypass operations on that part of the heart even as the organ continues to beat. The procedure can't be used on every patient, but it avoids the heart-lung machine's problems and can be considerably less expensive.

Though just a few years old, this technology is widely used. Gary Goodman, M.D., a cardiovascular surgeon at Detroit Medical Center, has operated with stabilizers more than 100 times.

"It allows us to perform (coronary bypasses), but without the heart-lung machine," he said. "It's still early, but it's really ushering in a new era of the way we do heart surgery, I suspect."

It will be years before we know the true impact of noninvasive procedures like the stabilizer, and no one can say what changes the future will bring. "You wonder where we're going to be 100 years from now," Goodman said. "They might look back at us in the 20th century and say, 'Boy, that was crude. They actually did surgeries for these problems. Imagine that.'"

SEEKING IMMUNITY

America's First Vaccine Arrived from England on a Silk Thread

by Linda Peterson

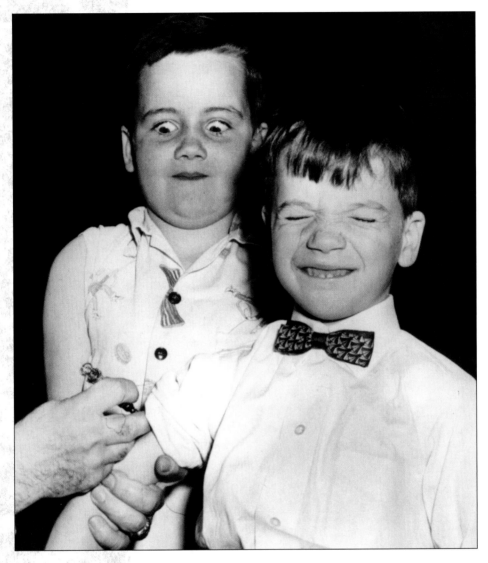

It only hurts if you look. *Philadelphia elementary-school children receive some of the first doses of Salk live polio vaccine in April 1955.* Source: Corbis-Bettmann

The history of childhood immunization in the United States stretches back to the earliest days of the republic. Two years after Englishman Edward Jenner published his carefully documented experiment using fluid from a cowpox lesion to successfully inoculate an 8-year-old boy against the far-deadlier smallpox, Harvard medical school professor Benjamin Waterhouse wrote Jenner to request vaccine material. Waterhouse used the vaccine, sent on a silk thread, to inoculate his 5-year-old son in July 1800.

President Thomas Jefferson followed these events with interest. He asked both men to send him vaccine; Jefferson used it to inoculate 18 members of his family.

It would be nearly 100 years before the next significant step in preventing disease through immunization. This time, the target was diphtheria, which, like smallpox, had washed in waves over the country since colonial times.

Combined Approach

In a March 1992 *New England Journal of Medicine* article "To End an Epidemic," UCLA School of Medicine professor Lawrence Kleinman, M.D., noted that diphtheria was the first infectious disease to be conquered on the basis of the principles of public health and microbiology.

Prominent late-19th century New York City physicians Abraham Jacobi, M.D., often called the father of American pediatrics, and social reformer August Caille, M.D., were instrumental in shaping that city's public-health response to the disease. Both men agreed with the findings of German scientists Theodore Klebs and Frederick Loeffler that diphtheria was a bacterial disease. Jacobi and Caille endorsed quarantine as a method to stem diphtheria's spread. Caille also spoke out for the need for better housing for the poor to alleviate the crowding that contributed to the spread of the disease.

The work of Klebs and Loeffler led first to a diphtheria antitoxin, which could lessen the disease's effect, and then to a preventive vaccine in 1918. The result: The average diphtheria death rate in 23 U.S. cities fell from 60 to 10 deaths per 100,000 between 1900 and 1930.

A tetanus vaccine soon followed. During World War II, immunization of troops virtually eliminated the disease as a result of war-related injuries. After the war, immunization of civilians became routine. The vaccine has proven to be almost ideal, providing long-lasting protection with few questions about its safety.

Safety Concerns

Unfortunately, the same cannot be said for the reputation of the pertussis (whooping cough) vaccine, which is now given to infants along with the diphtheria and tetanus vaccines in a "DPT" injection. As early as 1948, an article in *Pediatrics* linked the pertussis vaccine to neurological damage. A 1982 television report, "DPT: Vaccine Roulette," which some experts said was based on faulty research, dramatically increased the number of vaccine injury claims to DPT manufacturers. The resulting litigation costs drove some manufacturers out of the market, putting stress on the vaccine supply.

Congress responded with the National Vaccine Injury Compensation Program in 1986. The program was designed to serve as a no-fault insurance fund to compen-

sate for actual vaccine-related injuries. However, the program's first injury table listed some adverse reactions that had no accepted scientific data to back up a causal relationship.

The Institute of Medicine concluded: Vaccine-related risks are "extraordinarily small," and most purported adverse reactions are only coincidentally related by time, not by cause, to vaccination.

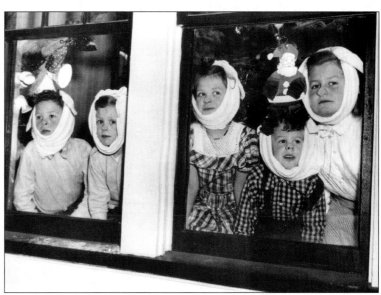

These siblings suffering from mumps watch their friends play in the snow on Christmas morning, 1948. Source: Corbis-Bettmann

One vaccine, however, does have an acknowledged link to an extremely serious, albeit rare, reaction. The Sabin oral polio vaccine—used more often than the earlier Salk injected vaccine because it costs less and is easier to administer—is linked to between eight and 10 cases a year of vaccine-caused polio. To address this issue, the polio vaccine recommendations call for the injected vaccine—which is a "killed virus" that carries no risk of causing polio—for the first two doses, and the oral vaccine for the final two doses. The rationale, said Jeanne Santoli, M.D., and Catherine DeAngelis, M.D., of Johns Hopkins University Medical School, is that the highest incidence of adverse reactions happens after the first vaccine dose.

A controversial vaccine for chickenpox became available in 1995. Questions include: Because childhood chickenpox is usually benign, do the immunization's benefits outweigh the costs? Because chickenpox is much more severe in adults than in children, if immunity fades will vaccinated children grow up to be susceptible adults? The benefits of the chickenpox vaccine have been judged to outweigh those concerns.

NO PLACE TO GO

*Crack Cocaine and HIV Created a Generation of Babies
Who Call the Hospital Home*

by Betty A. Marton

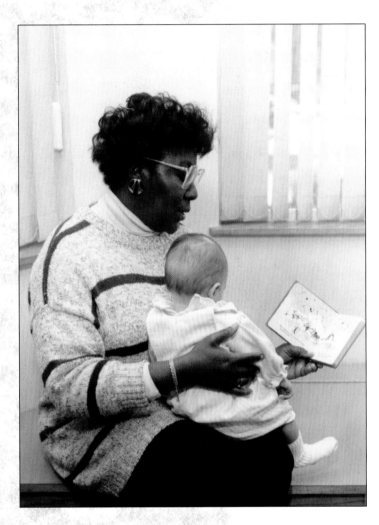

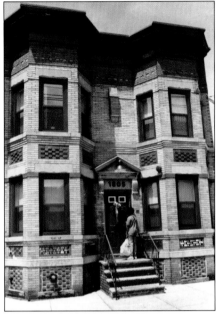

*It's story time (left) at Hudson Cradle in Jersey City, NJ,
where staff members care for infants who are abandoned or whose families are unable to care for them.
Before laws were enacted to set up such social-service
agencies, hospitals kept abandoned newborns until they
could be placed in foster care. Now, hospitals including
Jersey City Medical Center can send those so-called
boarder babies to facilities like Hudson Cradle, which is
housed in a converted brownstone (above).*

Photos courtesy of Hudson Cradle.

Julia's mother was in her mid-20s in 1991 when she
arrived at the Jersey City (NJ) Medical Center
(JCMC) about to deliver her fourth child. She had had
no prenatal care, admitted to using drugs, and told the
doctors, as well as she was able, just how often she had
used crack cocaine during the last few days.

Julia was born drug-addicted, underweight and with
medical problems. For 10 days, while she suffered
through withdrawal, her mother left the hospital,
returned once to visit her and then disappeared for good.

"She had already lost custody of her other three children because of her drug habits," said Nancy Floom,

assistant director for Social Work at JCMC. "She was
overwhelmed and helpless, like so many of the mothers
who come in here."

Left by her mother in the hospital, Julia became one of
many boarder babies—infants typically younger than 12
months who were cleared for discharge but have no one
to take them home.

Few Alternatives

A decade ago, boarder babies were straining the resources
of pediatric units, primarily in public hospitals. Although
babies have always been left behind in hospitals, their

numbers increased dramatically in the mid-1980s as families were fractured by rising rents, crack cocaine and HIV, wreaking havoc with inner-city lives. By 1991, up to 10,000 boarder babies stayed in 573 hospitals, from days after medical discharge to weeks or sometimes even months, at a cost of $22.3 million to $125 million.

"In 1989, we had between 30 and 50 babies in the hospital who stayed for up to a year before they were fostered out to care," said Jonathan Metsch, M.D., CEO of JCMC.

Before 1989, hospitals had few alternatives but to care for the babies left behind and many organized programs for volunteers to come and hold, rock and feed the babies.

"There weren't enough arms to go around," said Jill Seidler, who volunteered weekly at St. Luke's Hospital in New York City to help care for the infants there. "The medical staff had their hands full with sick children, but there were these other babies who just lay there crying because there was no one to pick them up."

Recognizing the crisis, Congress pulled together the Abandoned Infants Assistance Act in 1988 to fund social-service programs to get these babies out of the closed, windowless hospital nurseries and into alternative care.

"Most hospitals now automatically refer babies who test positive for drugs to child welfare services," said Amy Price, senior research associate at the Abandoned Infants Assistance Resource Center, a clearinghouse for programs established and funded through the Abandoned Infants Assistance Act.

Shifting the Problems

One of the programs funded by the act was Hudson Cradle, a converted brownstone with seven beds in Jersey City. Started by Metsch in 1991, Hudson Cradle provides care that focuses on the babies' health and development while working with family members and other care-givers to secure the infants' placement with suitable families. The center's residents are referred and supervised by New Jersey's Division of Youth and Family Services. Optimally, they stay for two months, but there are babies who begin to walk and talk before alternative placement is found.

In 1991, Julia became the first baby to leave JCMC for Hudson Cradle. When Hudson Cradle nurses and social workers reached out to Julia's extended family, they found an aunt who was willing to take her and who has adopted her. She is, Floom said, one of the few who end up with family members without ever having been in foster care.

Although the social issues related to drugs, HIV and homelessness that led to the epidemic of boarder babies in the mid-1980s still exist, the problems have shifted from hospitals to social-service agencies. Their efforts to intervene earlier to identify and work with families at risk, including mothers before they give birth, have resulted in a drop in the number of children who have entered the social-service system directly from the hospital to 9 percent in 1997 from 28 percent just a few years earlier.

"Social services help them get out of the hospital more quickly than before but that doesn't mean the problems have gone away," Floom said. "I have four babies here now just waiting for state intervention."

Staff members raised money to buy a "baby buggy" so their young charges could get some fresh air and sunshine. The tragedy of boarder babies has been exacerbated in the last decade because of increases in drug use, HIV infection and homelessness.

Photo courtesy of Hudson Cradle.

SHARING THE WEALTH

Philanthropies Were Major Influences in the Evolution of American Health Care

by Kevin Murray

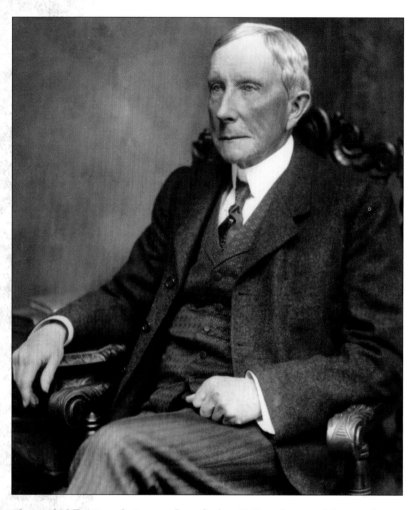

The Rockefeller Foundation was launched in 1913 with part of the vast fortune amassed by industrialist John D. Rockefeller Sr. The foundation's first targets were such diseases as malaria and hookworm that particularly affected poor southerners.   Source: Corbis-Bettmann

Beginning with the pioneering efforts of Thomas Bond, M.D., in 1751, health care philanthropy has dramatically influenced the development of hospitals. Bond, envisioning a hospital dedicated to the "reception and cure of poor sick persons," helped open the Pennsylvania Hospital of Philadelphia, the first general hospital in America. (*See* "Where the Evolution Began," on page 4.)

Early this century, major national philanthropic foundations pushed for the establishment of hospitals, particularly in rural areas, wrote Rosemary Stevens in her 1989 book *In Sickness and in Wealth*.

The Duke Endowment was among the first, and by far the largest, health care philanthropies. James Duke used his family's tobacco fortune to launch the Charlotte, NC-based endowment in 1924.

Duke indicated specifically how the endowment's funds should be used, said Gene Cochrane, vice president and director of health care for the endowment. He limited the not-for-profit hospital endowment geographically to the Carolinas.

"The early challenges of health care philanthropies clearly were how to get health care to the communities," Cochrane said.

Until about 1990, the vast majority of the endowment's funds helped hospitals build and expand, but in 1997, only 10 percent of the allocated funds supplied such capital.

"In the past, many hospitals looked at what is good for them as an institution or as an organization," Cochrane said. "I think that that still is important obviously, but increasingly hospitals are beginning to look more at what is good for their community."

The philosophical shift follows marketplace reality, he said.

"Grant requests are much more reflective of the type of issues that our hospitals are facing," Cochrane said. "For example, we have a number of requests for school-health programs, requests to help hospitals deal with the growing immigrant population, as well as lifestyle and wellness questions."

Duke endows hospitals that aim primarily to help those who lack access to health care. This includes helping hospitals create health care clinics and purchase mobile vans. Of the 161 hospitals the endowment currently supports, 12 percent to 15 percent of the endowment's approximate $23 million health care budget goes to the Durham, NC-based Duke Medical Center, Cochrane said.

Big Money, Massive Influence

Big philanthropies were responsible for shifts in hospital policy in the 1920s. They funded hospital standardization, consulting on a black veterans' hospital, organizing rural hospital demonstrations, and developing urban medical centers.

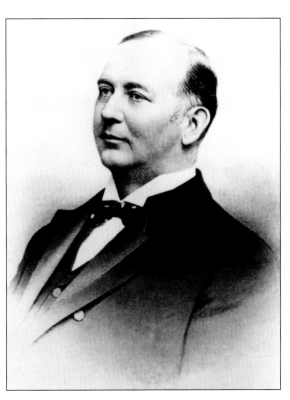

James Duke used his family's tobacco fortune to start the Duke Endowment in 1924. Until 1990, most of the endowment's funds helped build or expand hospitals, but changes in health care have led to a shift in the philosophy of giving for many philanthropies, including Duke. Source: Corbis-Bettmann

The New York City-based Rockefeller Foundation, another powerful philanthropic organization, began with a major health program in 1913.

"The concern was the control of disease that was particularly affecting the poor in the southern part of the United States; in particular, hookworm and malaria," said foundation Vice President Lincoln Chen, M.D.

"There was a flowering of the scientific revolution in medicine, and Rockefeller was very much the pioneer in believing that science needs to be harnessed for better health," Chen said.

"At that time, you had informal providers and doctors, but there was no standard curriculum, no training," Chen said. "Actually, doctors were very poorly paid and were not respected members of the community."

Public-health Impact

From 1913 to the late 1920s, the foundation endowed many of the leading medical schools, including Johns Hopkins and Harvard.

The foundation helped create schools of public health, including the first at Johns Hopkins in 1921, and another a year later at Harvard.

"Health has improved unbelievably over the last century," Chen said. "We've had more health gains globally in the last 40 years than we've had in the last 4,000 years."

"One of the future challenges [in health care philanthropy] will be how to share the fruits of modern civilization more broadly among the people of the United States."

Health care philanthropy now emphasizes global concerns, Chen said.

"People say that diseases don't need passports to travel," he said. "A disease that takes place anywhere in the world can reach the United States within 24 hours since there are over a million international travelers a day."

FAMILY TIES

Generations Follow One Another into Hospital Board Service

by Linda Peterson

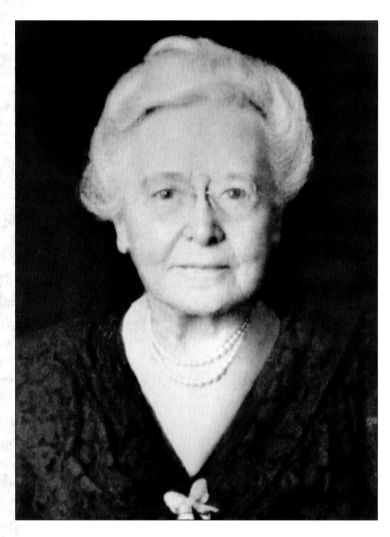

Margaret Roper Moss helped establish a visiting nurse service for poor mothers and their children in Norfolk, VA, in 1897. Moss' involvement in health care spanned 44 years and began a family tradition: her niece was a board member of Norfolk's Children's Hospital of the King's Daughters in the 1960s and great-niece Bruce Forsberg was a board member for 30 years, including six as chairwoman. Throughout the history of American hospitals, certain families have developed strong ties with institutions, and younger family members often have been encouraged to succeed their elders on boards of trustees.

Photo courtesy of the Children's Hospital of the King's Daughters.

William Saltonstall, third-generation member of the governing board of the New England Medical Center and its antecedent Boston Dispensary, has been, by all accounts, an exemplary trustee.

This despite the fact that he says he was drafted. "My uncle, Dick Saltonstall, who was serving as treasurer of the Boston Dispensary board of managers at the time, took me to lunch and said, 'Now, it is your turn.'"

William Saltonstall has earned "emeritus" trustee status after his long board service, from that draft lunch in the late 1950s and including his tenure as board chairman from 1979 to 1987.

He remains a frequent visitor to the medical center, says Joan Fallon, vice president for external affairs.

"If you walk around the hospital with him, he knows everyone." Fallon says. "People washing the floors, the nurses, the doctors, the technician—they all say, 'Hi, Bill.'"

Just like Grandma . . .

While the Saltonstall name is deeply rooted in New England history, it was Saltonstall's maternal grandmother, Eleanor Brooks, who began the Boston Dispensary board affiliation.

"The Boston Dispensary was located in an immigrant neighborhood," Saltonstall says. "One of their services was to help teach the mothers of neighborhood families about this country's food, since much of it was strange to them. My granny was in there ladling out soup."

Saltonstall says this with humor, but also proudly notes that today the New England Medical Center continues the tradition as an important research facility in the area of nutrition.

No Pressure

Bruce Forsberg became a board member of the Children's Hospital of the King's Daughters in Norfolk, VA, in 1967.

"I don't remember being pressured at all," she says, despite the fact that her great aunt was the founder of the hospital's predecessor organization—a visiting nurse service to the city's poor mothers and their children—and her mother was a hospital board member in the early 1960s.

Instead, Forsberg remembers thinking she "had died and gone to heaven" when she was able to accompany the visiting nurses on their rounds as a teenage member of a junior "circle" of the King's Daughters association in Norfolk.

The King's Daughters movement was founded in New York City in the late 1800s on the principle of service to others.

It was brought to Norfolk in 1886 by a group of young women who were members of a local Methodist church.

Ten years later, Norfolk had 14 King's Daughters circles.

Margaret Roper Moss—Forsberg's great-aunt—got the idea to strengthen their ability to help others by uniting them as the Norfolk City Union of the King's Daughters. Their first joint action was to establish the visiting nurse service in 1897, staffed by a single nurse who made her rounds by bicycle.

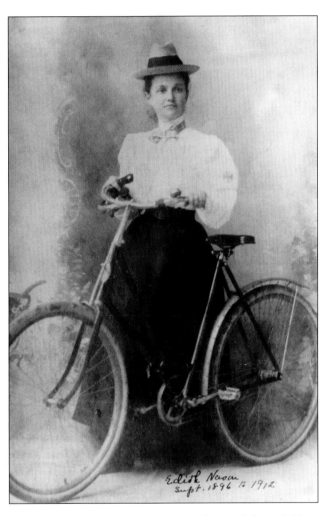

The visiting nurse service for poor mothers and their children in Norfolk, VA, established in 1897, was staffed by a single nurse who made her rounds on a bicycle.

Photo courtesy of the Children's Hospital of the King's Daughters.

For 44 years, Moss directed the King's Daughters circles in expanding the nursing service, adding neighborhood "health stations" and establishing a child health clinic. According to Forsberg's mother, Moss was both soft-spoken and businesslike—a particularly effective consensus-builder.

In the years following Moss' tenure, the King's Daughters realized their vision of building the region's only children's hospital. The hospital opened in 1961. Forsberg's mother, Elizabeth Roper Koolage, served on the board in its early years. Forsberg herself became a board member in 1967, staying for 30 years, six as board chairwoman.

Forsberg says that during her board chairmanship, her mother would often remark, "You're very much like your Aunt Marg."

Preserving Tradition

San Francisco's Chinese Hospital was founded in 1925 by 15 community groups in Chinatown to improve access to care for the city's Chinese immigrants.

Each group helped raise money to build the hospital, and each nominated a member to the hospital's board of trustees.

Early on, they recognized that language and cultural barriers got in the way of effective health care for the city's Chinese residents. So from the beginning, the hospital practiced Western medicine within the context of Chinese cultural traditions.

The Chinese Hospital's medical staff members are roughly 90 percent of Chinese descent. Of 110 active trustees, 17 are sons or daughters of parent physicians who served at the hospital, board chairman James Louie says.

AMERICA'S SAFETY NET

Public Hospitals Emerged from Humble—and Harrowing— Beginnings

by Jack Bess

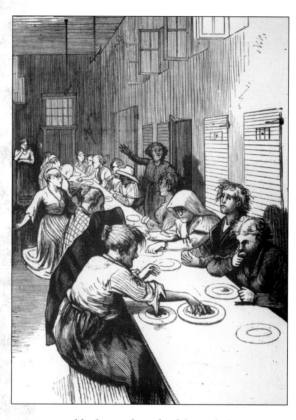

American public hospitals evolved from almhouses where ill paupers lived in grim, prison-like conditions with prostitutes, orphans, alcoholics, vagrants and criminals. Treatment was crude and overcrowding endemic. Philadelphia's Blockley almshouse was designated a hospital in 1835. The 1875 woodcut above depicts the dining room of the hospital's "insane asylum."

Source: Corbis-Bettmann

Public hospitals are health care's safety net—one that has been constructed over time strand by strand. Emerging as a clearly defined medical institution in the 19th century, public hospitals first had to shed most of the duties of the 18th century almshouse, only one of which was to care for the poor and sick. But even in their early incarnations, public hospitals had a mission that defines them to this day: They cared for people who had nowhere else to turn.

It took time for nascent public hospitals in such cities as New York, Philadelphia, Baltimore and Boston to shake off the traditions of the almshouse, an institution adopted from England in which criminals and debtors were put to work.

In early America, the almshouse clustered sick people, paupers, prostitutes, orphans, alcoholics and vagrants under the same roof. The atmosphere could be grim and prison-like. In the mid-18th century, the New York City almshouse, a forerunner of Bellevue Hospital, included "iron cages for psychiatric patients and whipping posts for slaves sent by their owners to be punished," according to *City Hospitals: The Undercare of the Underprivileged* by Harry K. Dowling, M.D.

The public hospital evolved from the almshouse out of physical necessity and a realization that these over-

burdened facilities had a significant medical purpose. And this purpose would best be served by a staff of medical professionals, while other almshouse functions—the orphanage, the jail and so on—would best be handled separately.

In 1816, the New York City almshouse-hospital averaged 200 patients but had a staff of just four: two visiting physicians who attended hospital patients twice a week and two interns who compounded all prescribed medications, gave post-operative care to surgical patients and oversaw the whole facility, including the penitentiary.

Overcrowding and filthy conditions that seemed to perpetuate illness persisted, as was described in an 1825 city report that "was as damning as words could make it," according to *The Bellevue Story* by Page Cooper. With heightened public awareness of the appalling conditions, the city appointed a board of visiting physicians and surgeons to the newly renamed Bellevue Hospital. This new board brought in medical students to accompany doctors on their rounds and began to peel off nonhospital functions. Male prisoners were separated in 1836, female prisoners in 1837, and the almshouse itself in 1848.

It was a pattern, Dowling notes, followed in such cities as Philadelphia, where the Blockley almshouse was designated a hospital in 1835 and nonhospital divisions were split away from 1874 to 1926, and Washington, DC, where the Washington Asylum became Gallinger Municipal Hospital in 1914 and other functions separated between 1903 and 1916.

Link to Medical Schools

As the public hospital evolved, so did the link between the institutions and medical schools. Just as almshouse hospitals provided a training ground for medical students, so did the emerging public hospitals, as they affiliated with newly formed medical colleges such as Philadelphia's College of Physicians and Surgeons (which opened in 1807) and New York University medical school (1841).

Public hospitals also became innovators in particular types of care. In the last half of the 19th century, Bellevue pioneered in several areas of care, Dowling wrote. The hospital established an outpatient department and an ambulance service, and founded a nurses' training school.

In addition, the new specialty services offered by public hospitals attracted "a fresh, vigorous group of doctors" eager to take part in rapidly developing fields of medicine, according to Dowling. Because private hospitals excluded patients with contagious diseases, public hospitals were forced to become specialists in treating

patients suffering from smallpox, scarlet fever, diphtheria and other ailments.

One of the strongest areas of specialty, Dowling pointed out, is pathology because many of the public hospital patients suffer from "unusual or advanced conditions less often seen in private hospitals."

Contemporary Challenges

That characteristic holds true for today's public hospitals, which provide certain services that some private hospitals see as too costly, said Chris Burch, executive vice president of the National Association of Public Hospitals & Health Systems (NAPH). These include neonatal intensive care, high-risk obstetrics and burn care.

In the 1990s, public hospitals face an array of challenges, including the rise in the number of uninsured patients and reductions in Medicaid coverage. They continue to serve people regardless of ability to pay.

According to NAPH statistics, 90 of the association's member hospitals reported in 1994 total staffed beds of 39,711 (an average of 442 per hospital), total admissions of 1,437,932 and total inpatient days of 10,912,944. Compared with the average private hospital in the 100 largest U.S. cities, the average NAPH hospital reported 30 percent more admissions, 39 percent more inpatient days and an occupancy rate (75 percent) that was 11 percent higher.

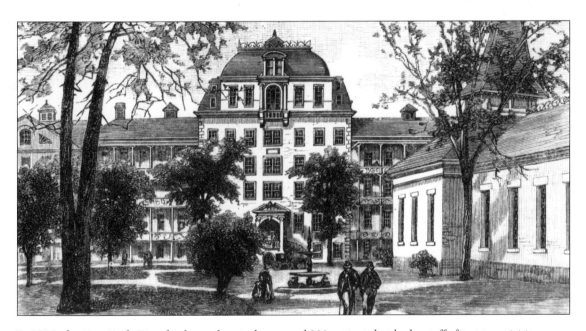

In 1816, the New York City almshouse-hospital averaged 200 patients but had a staff of just two visiting physicians who attended hospital patients twice a week and two interns. After a scathing 1825 city report, the New York City institution was renamed Bellevue Hospital, and its prison and almshouse functions separated from it over the next two decades. The engraving above shows Bellevue Hospital as it appeared in 1891.

Source: Corbis-Bettmann

LAST RIGHTS

As Ethicists Debate, Families and Doctors Confront Life-and-Death Decisions

by Betty A. Marton

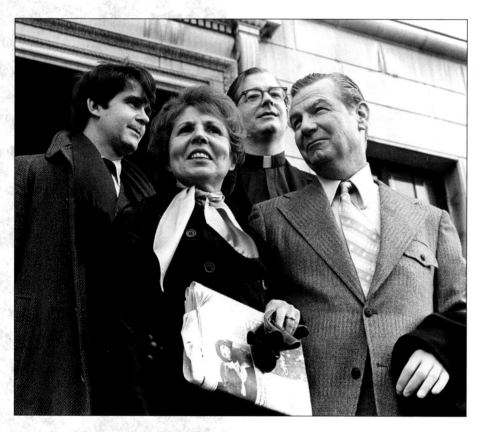

Julia and Joseph Quinlan leave New Jersey's Supreme Court building in Trenton in January 1976 with their lawyer and parish priest after justices heard appeal arguments in their attempt to end their comatose daughter's life. A lower court had refused permission to disconnect Karen (facing page), 21, from a respirator, which had been keeping her alive for more than nine months. The Quinlan case focused the debate over so-called futile care, a debate that continues to rage as medical technology advances. The New Jersey Supreme Court decided that Quinlan's 'right to privacy' included being removed from life support. Source: Corbis-Bettmann

In 1975, when Karen Ann Quinlan fell into a coma, she was eerily fulfilling two prophesies that she had made about herself: She was going to die young, she had told friends two years earlier, and she would make history.

Her second prediction came true when, after five months, Quinlan's parents asked doctors to remove their 21-year-old daughter from the ventilator that assisted her breathing. When they refused, Quinlan's parents took their case to the courts, eventually appealing it to the New Jersey Supreme Court, which decided that Quinlan's "right to privacy" included being removed from life support.

The Quinlan case brought into the public eye a debate that previously had been conducted largely behind closed doors, and in doing so, marked a new era in the ethical debate about end-of-life care.

"Quinlan does not mark the beginning of the movement to deal compassionately with terminally ill patients but, rather, the beginning of the movement's turn from the [scope] of patients, doctors, families, clerics and communities toward the sphere of the courtroom," writes M.L. Tina Stevens in American Cultural Politics and the Rise of Bioethics.

Another case that offered some guidelines for those wrestling with how to treat hopelessly ill patients was that of Baby Doe, which resulted in the 1984 amendment of the Child Abuse Prevention and Treatment Act stating that foregoing "medically indicated treatment" is a kind of medical neglect. That amendment also helped form the basis of the 1994 Baby K decision in which courts ruled that an anencephalic infant had the right to life-sustaining treatment even though there was no chance that she would ever gain consciousness.

The philosophical distance between the decisions regarding Karen Ann Quinlan—the right to the withdrawal of life-sustaining treatment—and those that won Baby K the right to have life-sustaining treatment some 20 years later represents a complete shift between physicians and families, according to Alexander Capron, professor of law and medicine at the University of Southern California, Los Angeles, and co-director of the Pacific Center for Health Policy and Ethics. Where physicians and hospitals were once reluctant to stop treatment and admit defeat, they now have incorporated the growing consensus of the larger community that aggressive treatment is often inappropriate.

"I think that what began to happen, particularly as technology advanced, is that the emotional sense shifted from a reluctance to stop treatment to a sense that continued treatment is an assault on a patient who isn't getting anything out of it and who's going to be dead anyway at the end of vigorous intervention," Capron said. "In many of the more contentious cases today, families and doctors have reversed their roles 180 degrees, with the families saying, 'Do anything possible,' and doctors saying, 'No, it's not worthwhile.'"

The American Medical Association's Council on Ethical and Judicial Affairs calls futile care an "inherently value-laden determination," but according to Jeffrey Botkin, M.D., associate professor of Pediatrics and Medical Ethics at the University of Utah in Salt Lake City, "Futile care needs to be looked at in terms of whether or not intervention will have an effect as well as whether or not an existence is worthwhile."

It also needs to be looked at in terms of the economic and social costs, according to the American Academy of Pediatrics Committee on Bioethics. Although the commit-

tee supports "individualized decision-making about life-sustaining medical treatment for all children, regardless of age," it also urges that "resource allocation decisions about which children should receive intensive care resources be made clear and explicit in public policy, rather than be made at bedside."

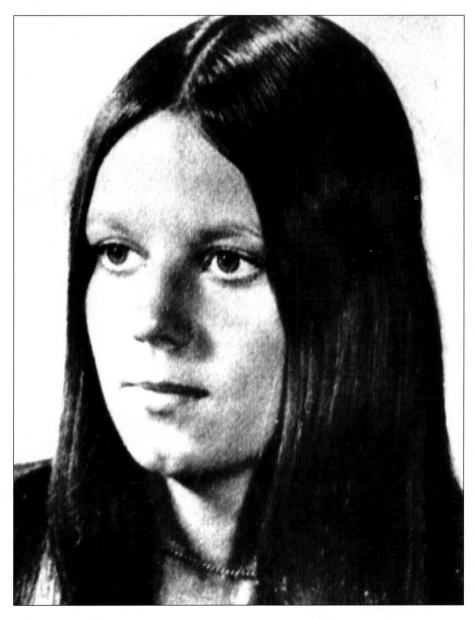

Source: Corbis-Bettmann

Botkin said the values agonized over in the Karen Ann Quinlan case are fundamentally the same as they were decades before and have been ever since.

"Technological advances and the courts, brought in as society's way of grappling with these issues, have made the debate stickier and more complex, but the values have stayed the same," Botkin said.

UNLIKELY ALLIES

Support for HMO Act Made for Strange Bedfellows

by Chris Larson

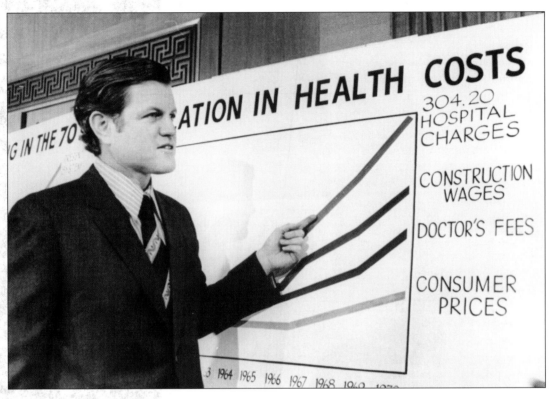

Uniting force. *The HMO Act united Republicans, Democrats, labor and industry. Sen. Edward M. Kennedy describes the need for reform during a 1971 briefing on health care inflation.*

Source: Corbis-Bettmann

When President Richard Nixon signed the HMO Act of 1973, a newspaper reported that his administration expected it to "have a major impact on medical care."

In 1970, there were fewer than 40 HMOs nationwide, serving about 2 percent of the population.

A dramatic change resulted from the HMO Act, and the unlikely coalition of ideologies and interest groups that helped push it through Congress and onto Nixon's desk.

To control rising health care costs, the Nixon administration turned to the relatively untested concept of managed care in 1971. In his 1972 State of the Union speech, Nixon said, HMOs "ought to be available everywhere so that families will have a choice." Proponents said HMOs would offer better care to more patients and be more cost-effective.

Prepaid group plans had been in operation on the West Coast since the early 1900s, but found breaking into new markets difficult.

Looking to Grow

"In many parts of the country, HMOs could not get a fair hearing," said Stuart Altman, professor of national health policy at Brandeis University.

As deputy assistant secretary for health policy at the U.S. Department of Health, Education and Welfare, Altman was one of the architects of the HMO Act. HMOs faced resistance from existing health plans, he said. With the act, "We were trying to open up the market for HMOs."

The bill, officially called the Health Maintenance Organization and Resource Development Act, designated $375 million in federal grants and loans to defray HMO start-up costs and specified what services an HMO had to offer to qualify for that money. It nullified some state laws that required a local medical board's approval before HMOs could be organized. Perhaps most importantly, it required companies with more than 25 employees to offer HMOs as an option in their health plan.

Several years of debate preceded the bill's passage. Many medical groups, including the American Medical Association, were opposed to the concept. In 1971, the AMA presented its views to the Senate: "The concept of the health maintenance organization has not yet been tested." It supported "further experimentation with HMOs," but felt that the bill was "a rather dangerous blank check to write . . . . There is an unfortunate tendency in this country to both over-promise and over-expect—especially where government programs are concerned."

Strange Bedfellows

Labor unions embraced the bill. Andrew J. Biemiller, director of the AFL-CIO's Department of Legislation, testified before Congress in 1971 that the group was "delighted with the rapidly growing interest in prepaid group practice." Unions disagreed with Nixon on many topics, he said, but "we are in complete accord on the importance of utilizing public funds to stimulate the development" of HMOs.

It was a classic case of strange political bedfellows.

"Most managed care was started and was viewed as socialized medicine, pure and simple," Altman said. "The supporters of managed care in the beginning were primarily the liberals. Then it was picked up in the early 1970s by the Republicans as market-oriented health care."

Within Congress, Democrats and Republicans argued mainly over the bill's finances: what specific programs an HMO had to offer, how much money would be available and whether funds would be allotted as grants or loans to start-up companies.

The final bill, sponsored by Democrats including Sen. Edward M. Kennedy (MA), passed in December 1973. Nixon signed it on Dec. 29.

The HMO industry generally was pleased with the law, but was concerned about restrictions. Shortly after the bill was enacted, an industry newsletter said requirements for open enrollment "might create competitive problems for HMOs." Looking back, Altman agreed. "What originally passed the Congress was so loaded down with requirements for what it took to be an HMO that it almost sunk the whole industry," he said. HMOs "just couldn't compete."

Early on, the government had envisioned 1,700 HMOs with 40 million members by 1976. In part because of the restrictions, it wasn't even close: by 1977, there were fewer than 7 million HMO members.

Congress amended the act in 1976, loosening the restrictions. HMOs began to grow faster, with 236 HMOs

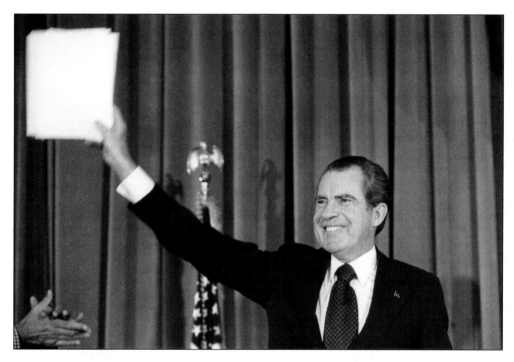

President Richard Nixon responds to hospital executives' approval by waving a copy of his 1974 AHA annual meeting speech.   Source: Corbis-Bettmann

and 9 million members in 1980.

The government then set a new goal of 442 HMOs and 19 million members by 1988. That proved much more reasonable, even conservative. In January 1988, more than 30 million people belonged to HMOs.

Some 650 HMOs exist nationwide today and enrollment tops 60 million.

"It's been an amazingly successful program," Altman said. "Without it, I doubt whether the managed care revolution of the '80s and '90s would ever have happened."

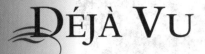

DÉJÀ VU

Road to Reform Runs Politicians in Circles

by Jack Bess

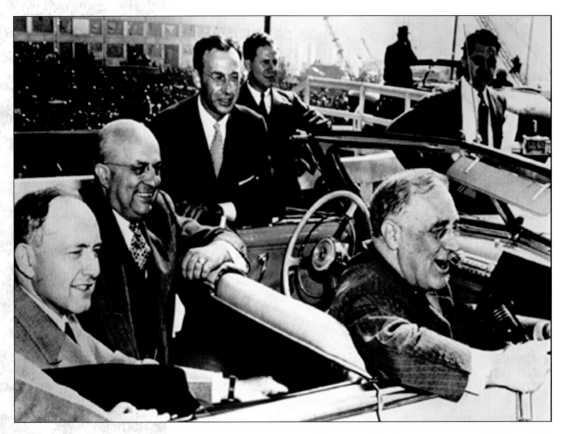

President Franklin Roosevelt addresses Kaiser shipyard workers in Portland, OR, in 1942, with (from left) Oregon Gov. Charles Sprague, Henry J. Kaiser and his son Edgar Kaiser. Early in his administration, Roosevelt's Social Security Act had included a recommendation that federal officials consider a government health insurance program. The outcry, especially from physicians, that any such proposal was akin to socialism and communism, caused Roosevelt to back off the suggestion so as not to imperil the rest of the Social Security bill. Henry Kaiser started a hospital for builders of the Grand Coulee Dam in the 1930s. In 1945, he offered open enrollment to the public in his health care system, which by 1995 had become the nation's oldest and largest not-for-profit HMO. Source: AP/Wide World Photo

Some of Washington's fiercest political debates have centered on health care. Political heat has fueled these fires, but unresolved problems confront each administration and Congress: What role, if any, can the government play in guaranteeing access to care without taking a step on the road to socialized medicine?

Amid the New Deal programs created by Franklin D. Roosevelt's White House, the Social Security Act recommended that federal officials consider concepts for group practice and health coverage, including a government health insurance program. A blue-ribbon panel called the Committee on the Costs of Medical Care made the proposal in 1934, after it found that family income determined Americans' access to care.

Roosevelt Backs Down

Doctors' anxiety ran sky-high. An editorial in the *Journal of the American Medical Association* stated that the committee's ideas would lead to "the destruction of private practice." *JAMA's* editors called the proposal akin to socialism and communism and said it would incite revolution.

Political opposition mounted, and Roosevelt, worried about the fate of the Social Security bill, backed off.

Still, notions of a government-sponsored health care plan persisted. In the 1940s, bills proposing compulsory government insurance were introduced in Congress by Democrats Rep. John Dingell Sr. (MI) and Sens. Robert Wagner (NY) and James Murray (MT), who were inspired by Britain's 1942 social security act.

Truman's Plan

President Harry S. Truman took up the crusade in November 1945. His agenda included broadening Social Security to include compulsory insurance, funded by a payroll tax. Bills containing Truman's plan died in Congress, but the ideas didn't wait long for resurrection. In 1949, the newly re-elected Truman repeated his call. His administration projected that the program could be financed with a 3 percent payroll tax, 1.5 percent each from the employer and employee. Educated guesses put the plan's cost anywhere from $3 billion to $8 billion annually.

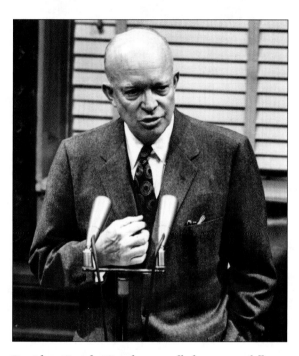

President Dwight Eisenhower called unsuccessfully for a $100 million government funding to encourage private companies to experiment with more comprehensive insurance policies.

Source: Corbis-Bettmann

Some argued that climbing medical costs and inadequate voluntary health plans were dooming those who "can't afford to live," as Murray put it. "The relation between money and life—between wealth and health—is direct and deadly."

Such critics as Sen. Robert Taft (R-OH) warned that the Truman plan would make all doctors government employees. Others, such as AHA President John H. Hayes, argued that the emerging success of voluntary Blue Cross plans proved that Americans could provide for themselves without "a cumbersome federal scheme of compulsion."

Truman backed off in 1951, about the time that federal officials began discussing a new idea called "health reinsurance." It was a concept that President Dwight D. Eisenhower would make the backbone of his health program in 1954.

Ike Relies on Private Market

Eisenhower's unsuccessful proposal called for a $100 million government fund that would be used to reinsure private companies that offered expanded benefits to individual purchasers. If a private insurer had to pay more than a given amount in sick claims, the *Congressional Digest* explained, that company could, if it reinsured with the government, be reimbursed for part of its loss.

Proponents of reinsurance said the policy would stimulate private companies to experiment with more comprehensive policies, broadening coverage to include heart disease and cancer. But such opponents as the U.S. Chamber of Commerce countered that broadening coverage would lead insurers into huge losses that would require large federal subsidies.

Social Security Broadened

Congress continued to grapple with reform. The Kerr-Mills Act amended Social Security in 1960, increasing federal grants to states for welfare recipients' care. Early in 1961, President John F. Kennedy called for extending Social Security benefits to cover hospital and nursing-home care.

Although that bill was defeated, other proposals followed quickly. Labor and welfare groups and such legislators as Sen. Hubert Humphrey (D-MN) noted that senior citizens were enjoying longer lives and that advances in technology were driving up the cost of care—factors that created a crushing burden for the uninsured. On the other side, the AMA warned of "political opportunists . . . dedicated to the destruction of medicine as a free institution," and Sen. Barry Goldwater (R-AZ) claimed that expanding welfare would erode Americans' obligations to care for family members.

The Medicaid and Medicare legislation that eventually passed in 1965 was a compromise incorporating elements of three bills, including a Republican-sponsored measure that contained the American Medical Association's proposal for private insurance carriers to offer a separate voluntary plan that covered physicians' services to the elderly.

LABOR PAINS

Legal and Workplace Changes Fostered Unions

by Chris Larson

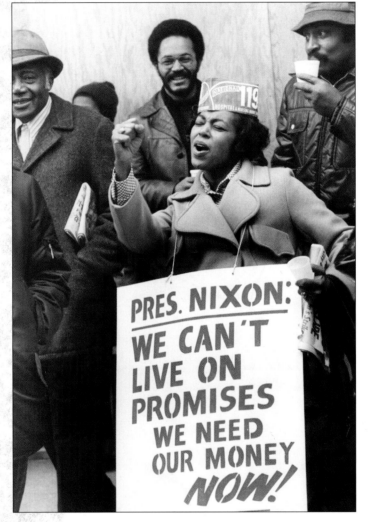

A hospital worker joins more than 30,000 technical, service and maintenance workers who walked off their jobs in November 1973 at 48 New York City hospitals. Under pressure from unions, Congress amended Taft-Hartley in 1974 to allow workers at private, not-for-profit hospitals to organize and strike but with considerable restrictions. Source: Corbis-Bettmann

Though never completely shut out, labor unions have had a tough time getting into hospitals. Circumstances and laws kept hospitals union-free for much of this century. It's only very recently that economics and court rulings have converged to make hospitals an easier mark for union organizing.

Unions in every industry promise their members improved wages and benefits. That argument has never worked well in hospitals, according to Kevin Scanlan, vice president of human resource services at the Metropolitan Chicago Healthcare Council. "The health care industry already offers extremely competitive compensation and benefits." Unions thus lose one of their main selling points.

Workers have been organizing in the United States since at least the Industrial Revolution, yet it wasn't until 1916 that health care workers first formed a union, at Chicago's Cook County Hospital. The next two decades saw organizing and strikes at just a few other public hospitals.

The National Labor Relations Act, passed in 1935, guaranteed workers in most industries, including health care, the right to organize and strike. Labor unions saw huge increases in their membership over the next decade. Union drives were successful at some hospitals—including the first at a private hospital, in San Francisco in 1941—but most of that growth came from the manufacturing industry, not health care.

Hospitals wanted to keep it that way. Arguing that they were a unique industry—made up mostly of not-for-profit, charitable entities—and essential to the community, health care organizations lobbied Congress to change the law.

Congress did so in 1947 with the Taft-Hartley Act, which restricted union organizing. The new law excluded employees of private not-for-profit hospitals from National Labor Relations Act protection.

Unions Go State to State

Health care unions weren't banned by the law; each state could pass its own laws regarding unions in hospitals.

So labor unions and groups like the American Nurses Association had to try to change laws state by state. They had the most success in the Northeast.

Responding to pressure from unions, Congress amended Taft-Hartley in 1974. Workers at not-for-profit hospitals once again could join unions and strike. The bill included significant restrictions; most notable was the 10-day notice unions must provide before a health care strike.

The bill immediately resulted in more labor activity. Between 1974 and 1978, health care institutions faced more than 1,000 union elections. Unions won just over half of them, AHA statistics show.

Organizing slowed in the 1980s. Then, in April 1989, the National Labor Relations Board ruled that health care workers would be classified into eight collective-bargaining units. Each unit would be very specific: maintenance workers in one, for instance, and registered nurses in another.

Earlier rules allowed just four health care bargaining units, resulting in large groups of employees with wide-ranging job duties that unions found hard to organize.

Labor unions were thrilled by the change. It's much easier to win a union election if everyone in the group does the same work. Unions nationwide made plans for intense hospital organizing efforts. One union official said at the time that the ruling would "open up possibilities that didn't exist before."

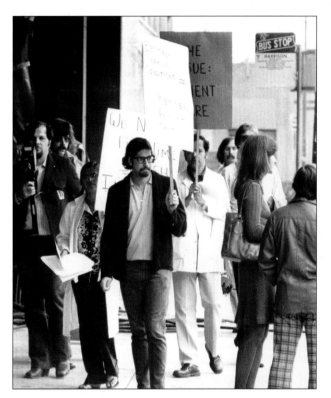

Medical residents and interns refused a court order to end their walkout against Chicago's Cook County Hospital in October 1975. It was at Cook County Hospital that the first health care union was formed in 1916.

Source: Corbis-Bettmann

Hospitals didn't like those possibilities. The AHA immediately sued to have the ruling overturned, saying in a 1990 memo that it "not only would disrupt the delivery of health care, but also would significantly increase [hospital costs] at a time when escalating health care expenses are a pressing national problem."

Ultimately, the Supreme Court didn't rule on the merits of the case, but in 1991 declared unanimously that the National Labor Relations Board (NLRB) had the authority to make the ruling.

At the same time, changes in the health care field put intense financial pressures on hospitals, Scanlan said. Employees had to face the unfamiliar prospect of reduced job security.

Buoyed by the Supreme Court decision, unions began to organize in earnest. They targeted more specific groups of workers, and with a new appeal: Benefits and wages might still be competitive, but unions help workers keep their jobs.

It's too soon to tell the final outcome of the NLRB ruling.

Each side claims victories. Unions have won some recent drives, but lost others by as much as a 3-to-1 vote.

The only certainty is that union drives will continue.

"I think there's going to be more unionization activity, at a level we've never seen before," said Rick Wade, AHA senior vice president of communications.

Employees at all levels, from security guards and clerical staff to RNs and physicians, will be asked to consider unions in coming years, Wade said.

But that doesn't necessarily bode ill for hospitals.

"We're seeing some unions today that are far less adversarial, more in partnership with the hospital," he said. "Hospitals and unions are saying, 'We need a different kind of working relationship than we've had.' We're beginning to see some of that happen."

IF YOU BUILD IT . . .

Millions in Federal Money Prompted a Hospital Building Boom

by Jack Bess

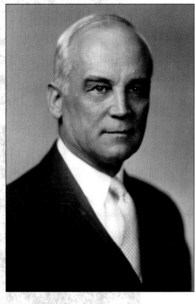

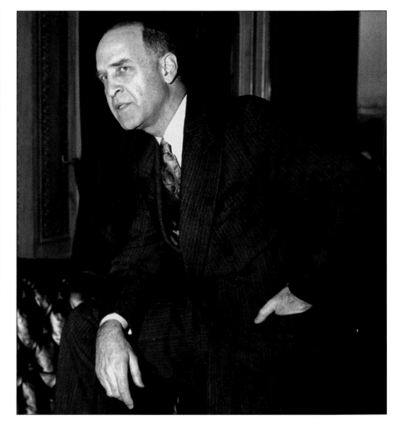

Legislation introduced in 1946 by U.S. Sens. Harold Burton and Lister Hill (above left and right, respectively) created a five-year program to provide $75 million a year in federal matching grants to states to build hospitals and medical centers and $3 million for all states to inventory their health facilities.

Source: The U.S. Senate Historical Office

Imagine a time when U.S. hospitals had waiting lists of inpatients. Overcrowded urban hospitals weren't unusual in the years of World War II. In New York City, some people were checking into hospitals for ailments as minor as the common cold.

At least one contemporary press account quoted a lament that "beds scarcely have time to cool off between patients."

The problem of inadequate hospital capacity actually predated the 1940s, but solving it was postponed by the Great Depression and World War II. Waging a world war created a voracious need for building materials for military purposes, and thus brought new hospital construction in the U.S. to a near-standstill.

The stage was set for a post-war hospital building boom, made possible in 1946 by legislation called the Hospital Survey and Construction Act, better known as the Hill-Burton Act. Sponsored by U.S. Sens. Lister Hill (D-AL) and Harold Burton (R-OH), the legislation created a five-year program in which $75 million in matching grants would be provided annually to states to build hospitals in underserved areas.

In return for accepting Hill-Burton funding, hospitals had to assure that their facilities would be available to the community at large in perpetuity and agree to provide charity care. These requirements were un-specified until the 1960s and 1970s when a series of court cases and regulatory actions redefined hospitals' uncompensated care obligations. Although the charity care requirements were limited to 20 years and the last Hill-Burton funding was awarded in the mid-1970s, some hospitals are still fulfilling their obligations because of regulatory actions.

The law also appropriated $3 million for all states to inventory their health facilities. For the first time, the nation would have a comprehensive picture of where the need for hospitals was most urgent, and each state would have a planning process for meeting that need.

While hospital growth thrived in the early 20th century, reaching a total of 6,850 hospitals by 1928, that expansion came to a halt with the stock market crash in 1929. Economic hardship contributed to the closing of nearly 800 hospitals from 1928 to 1938.

Hospital building didn't stop entirely. The Roosevelt administration launched public-works programs that included remodeling and building hospitals. Even with the war effort devouring construction material in the 1940s, a few hospitals were built in areas with high populations of defense workers.

By 1944, health officials were anticipating a flowering of hospitals in a postwar world. In October of that year, the Commission on Hospital Care was organized under the sponsorship of the AHA and with assistance from the U.S. Public Health Service. Surveying each state, the commission concluded that more than 195,000 new general-hospital beds were needed. Federal funding was key to the effort. The bill found strong support in Congress. As some legislators pushed for national health insurance, Hill-Burton backers such as Sen. Robert Taft argued that the measure would give states the ability to make their own plans rather than allowing the "federal government to take over the entire medical care program of the United States."

President Harry S. Truman signed the bill on Aug. 13, 1946. Shortly thereafter, Surgeon General Thomas Parran, M.D., said priority would be given to areas with large minority populations and rural communities where health facilities were nonexistent or outdated.

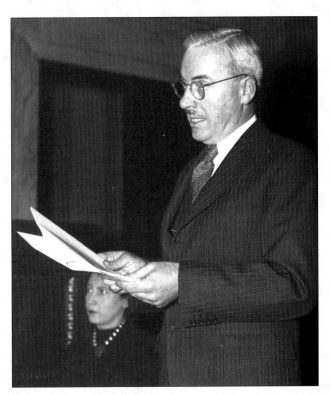

Shortly after Congress passed the bill and President Harry Truman signed it into law, Surgeon General Thomas Parran, M.D., said priority would be given to areas with large minority populations and rural communities. The Hill-Burton program later was extended and enlarged to provide building grants for such facilities as nursing homes, diagnostic and treatment centers, rehab centers and chronic disease hospitals. By the program's 20th anniversary, Hill-Burton accounted for an estimated 349,318 inpatient beds.

Source: Corbis-Bettmann

By December 1947, the federal government had 53 applications for new hospitals, about 70 percent of which were from towns with fewer than 5,000 residents.

One of the early grant recipients in 1947 was Mount Vernon, IL, an industrial town of about 21,000 residents, which received nearly $388,000 to build a 100-bed hospital. Its existing facility, a century-old hospital, had an operating room with buckling brick walls, a shack for storing records, an old cabinet that served as a clinical laboratory and an emergency room that originally was intended as a conference room.

Many of the new hospitals used as a construction blueprint the Public Health Service's "Study on Hospital Design." The study's significance, according to "The Hospital: A Social and Architectural History" by John D. Thompson and Grace Goldin, was that "For the first time, an attempt was made to standardize hospital measurements. Hospitals had been built with 24-inch doors that would not take a hospital bed. No one ever asked what would be done to get the patient out of such wards in case of fire."

A key concept in the new hospital designs was to create a more "human" setting that would enhance patients' comfort and privacy. The Health Service guidelines even suggested that a new hospital site should be chosen with an eye toward making sure that every patient's room would receive sunlight during at least part of the day.

The Hill-Burton program was extended in subsequent years to provide grants for building nursing homes, diagnostic and treatment centers, rehab centers and chronic disease hospitals. By 1966, which marked the program's 20th anniversary, Hill-Burton accounted for nearly 8,200 construction and expansion projects that provided an estimated 349,318 inpatient beds.

REMOTE POSSIBILITIES

North Carolina Pioneered Health Care Programs for Rural Americans

by Matthew Weinstock

Providing care to the nation's most isolated areas has never been easy. But one state—perhaps more than any other—has viewed rural health care not as an insurmountable crisis but as an opportunity to find community-based solutions.

Several experts say that North Carolina forged a path for other states to follow. As one put it, "North Carolina learned to put theory into practice."

To understand how far North Carolina has come, it's important first to realize how bad conditions were.

As early as 1909, policymakers, educators and health care providers were calling attention to the state's lack of access to care. While there were some success stories—Robeson County in 1912 became the first county in the state to hire a full-time health director—the plight of rural health care did not garner much attention.

In fact, the public at large did not start paying close attention to rural health care until the 1940s.

While thousands of men and women were called to serve in World War II, relatively few North Carolinians actually saw any action. The state had the highest medical rejection rate for draftees of any state in the union.

The causes ranged from poor nutrition to bad or unavailable medical care, according to Thomas Ricketts, director of the North Carolina Rural Health Research Program. It is important to note, Ricketts said, that most of North Carolina was considered rural at that time—

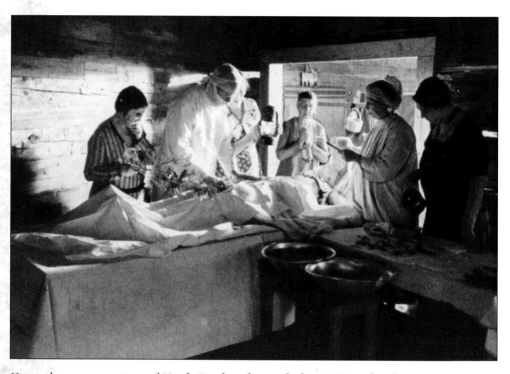

Hospitals were scarce in rural North Carolina during the late 1800s and early 1900s. Doctors sometimes had to perform surgery on kitchen tables in their patients' homes, as in the photo above. Source: NC Division of Archives

according to the 1940 census, 72.7 percent of the population lived in rural areas.

All Health Care Is Local

In the next 40 years, the state launched a number of innovative and ambitious projects focusing on rural health care.

A guiding principle in these programs was that local communities could best deal with the crisis. The citizenry pushed for more local involvement in health care programs, said Jim Bernstein, head of North Carolina's office of rural health.

Three of the most significant developments that helped shape the future of rural care nationwide occurred in the late 1960s and early 1970s, a time when access to care was at an all-time low. North Carolina ranked 43rd of the 50 states in the ratio of physicians to population. Worse yet, it ranked 46th in the ratio of medical students to population.

To turn the tide, East Carolina Medical School was founded in the predominately rural and poor eastern part of the state in 1967. It was the state's fourth medical school.

Just as important as the new medical school, North Carolina established the Area Health Education Centers (AHEC) program.

Each AHEC center—run by its own local board—had a relationship with a major medical school and supported training at the local level. These centers served as a model for AHEC centers across the nation.

Today, they continue to be critical to ensuring the equitable distribution of health care providers, Ricketts said.

Harnessing the Horses

Educating more doctors and coordinating their placement is all well and good, Bernstein said, but rural communities still faced an immediate need for quality care.

So, in 1973 lawmakers gave birth to the Office of Rural Health and Resource Development—the first such state office in the country. The new office helped rural communities increase access to care.

"People were crying out for help. So we told them to organize and form nonprofit organizations," Bernstein explained. "If they did that, we would provide funds and technical assistance to build health centers."

Also, the office pushed a novel and highly controversial idea: use mid-level practitioners to administer care.

"Medical students take years to finish school," Bernstein noted. "We could get a nurse practitioner or physician assistant to provide primary care in about a year."

Over time, the office changed its focus to recruiting

physicians. The doctor-to-population ratio has decreased nearly 40 percent since 1974 when there was one physician for every 3,200 residents. In 1995, the most recent year for which such data is available, there was one physician for every 1,858 residents.

While access to care in rural North Carolina has improved, there is a long way to go, Bernstein said, adding that the best solutions use the entire community. "We have the horses, we just have to harness them—the schools, social services, the hospitals. We have to get everyone working together," he said.

During the next few years, North Carolina will try out another innovative idea, this time with its Medicaid managed care program. Bernstein's office plans to fund two demonstration projects next year, both establishing networks made up of health care providers, schools, social services and other local entities that will run managed care programs for a select number of Medicaid recipients.

"We will give them the funds and hold them accountable," he said. "The hardware is out there, we just need all the pieces to fit together."

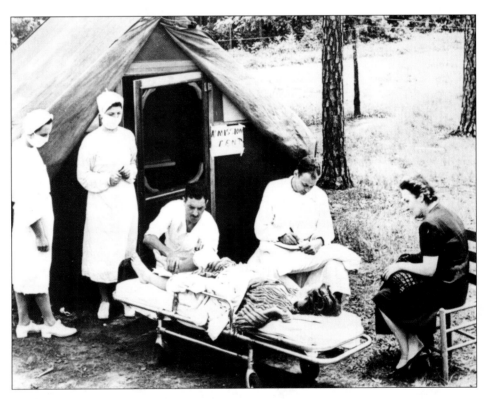

In the 1940s, North Carolina began to focus on rural health care, implementing innovative programs and policies that soon were copied by other states. In response to a 1944 polio epidemic, a camp in Hickory, NC, was converted into an emergency polio hospital within a matter of days. The hospital became known as the "Miracle of Hickory."

Source: NC Museum of History

On a Mission from God

Nuns' Healing Spirit Tamed the Frontier

by Philip Dunn

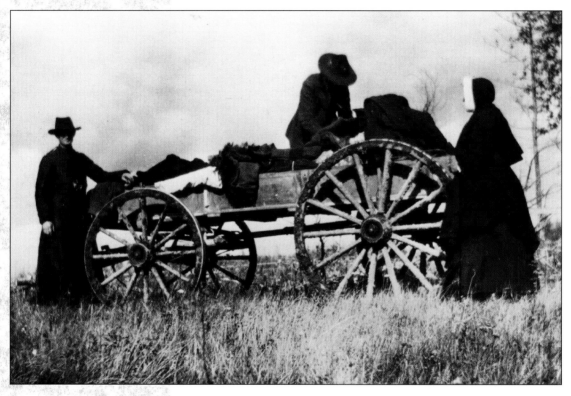

Catholic missionaries, including Sister Chiasson of the Sisters of Providence, move supplies for American Indian missions in Idaho and Montana, around 1900. Photo courtesy of Sisters of Providence Archives, Seattle.

In 1866, Galveston, TX, Bishop Claude Marie Dubuis appealed for help in establishing hospitals and orphanages. Three nuns from Lyons, France, responded.

The Civil War had just ended, and Texas still had a reputation as a lawless land. Unlike most places on the frontier, Catholicism was well-established there, representing the Mexican-Catholic tradition, descended from the Spanish, rather than the Irish, French or Italian traditions that were more common in America's eastern cities. However, "settlers," whether they shared a common religion or not, were viewed with suspicion.

The three nuns, members of the Congregation of the Sisters of Charity of the Incarnate Word, arrived in Galveston, an unfamiliar place with a strange language. An epidemic of yellow fever soon hit, and one of the sisters died.

"They were facing such tough odds," says historian Christopher J. Kauffman, author of *Ministry & Meaning: A Religious History of Catholic Health Care in the United States.*

"The fact is this was very much a man's world out on the frontier," Kauffman says. "For these women to go out like that and establish missionary health care facilities is quite a stunning achievement."

As children, Americans learned that the West was settled by heroic soldiers doing battle with marauding Indians (that legend has been revised by historically more accurate and sensitive accounts). But while men were off being cowboys, it was religious women—particularly nuns—who were caring for the sick.

In their missionary zeal, nuns from several orders went west in the 19th century to establish hospitals for railroad workers and miners.

Their work paid off. Catholic nuns established the first hospitals in such frontier outposts as Chicago, Milwaukee, Boise, Salt Lake City, San Antonio, Seattle and Portland.

The Interfaith Model

The story of the Sisters of Charity of the Incarnate Word is, in many ways, typical. Sent by their church, they went to a strange and dangerous place, with little help from religious men.

It took a particularly strong woman, both physically and spiritually, to do that kind of work.

"The reputation of the sisters goes back to the origins of health care in Europe," Kauffman says. "The sister had been identified as the principal care-giver in the Catholic community. But on the frontier it was very difficult, because they could be the only women around."

Despite the hardships in Texas, the nuns persevered. By 1869, their number grew to 12, and they began work to establish a hospital in San Antonio. In 1885, with their numbers still growing, they helped establish the Missouri Pacific Railroad Hospital in Forth Worth.

In addition to being hearty, the nuns were resourceful. Because (with the exception of the Southwest) there were generally few Catholics on the frontier, Catholic care-givers often worked with those outside the church—from other religious quarters and from other community institutions and employers—to establish hospitals and raise funds.

Typical is the story of Mother Joseph Pariseau of Montreal, who led five Sisters of Charity of Providence to Vancouver, British Columbia, arriving Dec. 8, 1856.

Pariseau helped build Vancouver's first hospital two years later with the help of the town's Jewish and Protestant residents. It became one of the first models of cooperation among religious groups to accomplish collectively what would have been impossible alone.

"They were depending on funds from the entire community, so in a sense these were community hospitals," Kauffman says. "Although in many instances the Catholic hospitals were the first in their areas, they relied upon people of good will from all religious traditions."

Mother Pariseau went on to lead her order in establishing hospitals in Seattle and Portland. By the time she died in 1902, there were 250 nuns in Oregon, Washington and Vancouver, and nuns from other orders had established hospitals in Tacoma and Aberdeen, WA. Although

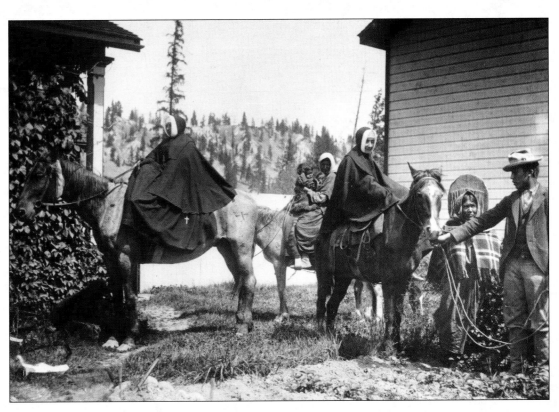

Because money was tight, some Catholic health care leaders went on "begging tours" to raise funds. In this photo, nuns from Portland, OR, and guides embark on a begging tour to raise money for a new hospital in Kootenay, British Columbia.   Photo courtesy of Sisters of Providence Archives, Seattle.

Mother Pariseau is renowned for her building feats (the American Institute of Architects recognizes her as the first architect of the Northwest), she initially made her mark by establishing hospitals.

"It took a rather resilient person to be able to withstand the hard times," Kauffman says. "But the challenge is invigorating. It's stimulating work. They didn't join for comfort."

FEAR THE WORST

Even the Best Contingency Plans Are Vulnerable to Disaster

by Jack Bess

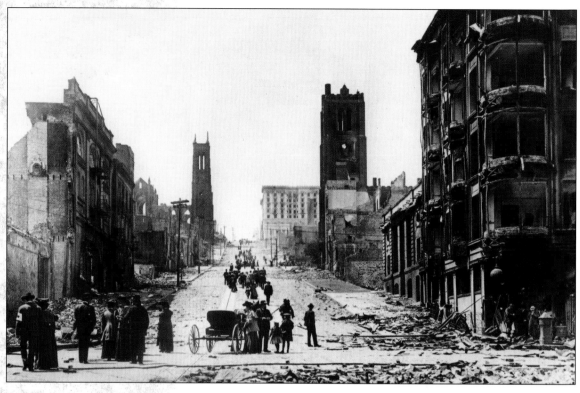

The "San Francisco Horror." A view of California Street west from Kearney following the 1906 San Francisco earthquake. Source: Corbis-Bettmann

Unlike the proverbial generals always preparing to fight the previous war, hospital officials keep one eye on history and the other on the future in preparing their disaster plans.

Bitter experience has provided some guidelines for anticipating such calamities as earthquakes, tornadoes and hurricanes.

One of the most trying of all disasters was the 1906 earthquake and subsequent fire dubbed the "San Francisco Horror."

Striking in the early morning of April 18, the earthquake dealt punishing blows to the city's infrastructure and left tens of thousands homeless. More than 28,000 buildings were destroyed.

The fires that raged, ultimately wiping out 4.7 square miles of the city, set the stage for the dramatic evacuation of St. Mary's Hospital.

With flames approaching, St. Mary's doctors and nursing sisters launched an evacuation plan drawn up just hours earlier.

"As our patients were removed from their beds, the mattresses were thrown through the windows, and the patients were carried to waiting trucks," the hospital matron, Mother Euphrasia, later recalled.

Just as the fire reached the hospital, showering staff members with red-hot cinders, someone handed a nurse a small baby, the last evacuee. "Nobody knew to whom it belonged," Mother Euphrasia said.

The escape from the city is described in *The San Francisco Earthquake* by Gordon Thomas and Max Morgan Witts. "Surgical dressings, trolleys, instruments, [and] drugs were dumped into laundry boxes, loaded onto trucks, and rushed to the Pacific Mail dock where the river paddle steamer *Medoc* had been berthed all afternoon," they wrote. The riverboat had been transformed into a floating hospital.

About 150 patients were aboard, lying on mattresses that stretched across the decks. Those who died were laid inside a lifeboat. The Sisters of St. Mary's later set up a tent hospital near Golden Gate Park.

Although the 1906 earthquake led health care officials to develop contingencies for future disasters, even the most finely tuned plans are vulnerable to one-of-a-kind circumstances.

The 1989 earthquake that rocked the San Francisco Bay area caused a stretch of Interstate 880 to collapse, killing dozens of motorists. As one physician told *The Los Angeles Times*, "No amount of medical preparedness can address the problem of collapsed concrete."

Human behavior following a disaster is another wild card that can challenge the emergency medical system.

After a tornado sliced through Texas and Oklahoma in 1947, killing an estimated 132 people and injuring 1,305, local hospitals were overrun not only by the injured but by thousands of uninjured people as well.

"The hospitals became very quickly a sort of madhouse, with everybody running in to see what was happening," according to a 1958 account, *Tornadoes Over Texas*.

People sometimes react to emergencies in ways that are unexpected but, in retrospect, completely logical. Hospital staffs learned some "interesting things" in the 1994 Northridge, CA, earthquake, said Roger Richter, senior vice president of professional services for the California Healthcare Association.

Hospital "staff rushed in to provide assistance in the emergency rooms, but the patients didn't show up until some time later," Richter said. "Patients who were injured

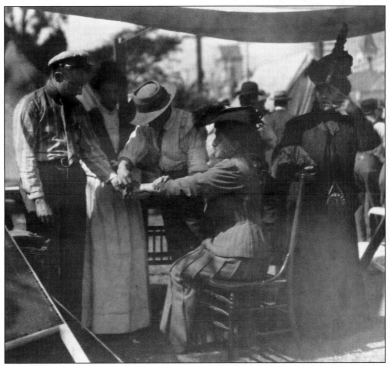

After the 1906 San Francisco earthquake, officials of the destroyed St. Mary's Hospital quickly set up a tent hospital in Golden Gate Park.

Source: Library of Congress/Corbis-Bettmann

wanted to make sure their families were safe and their possessions were secured, then they came in with their cuts and scratches and broken bones." But by then, many staff members had left to check on their own families, leaving a skeleton crew to face the crush.

While hospital buildings largely withstood the Northridge quake, some facilities were forced to shut down because of serious damage to water mains, oxygen lines and power systems. When power failed at Northridge Hospital Medical Center, nurses in the neonatal ICU unhooked babies from lifeless machines and carried them down darkened stairwells. Medical staff tended to patients in a makeshift emergency room in the parking lot.

In the aftermath, the state passed a law requiring all general and acute care hospitals to be retrofitted to the minimum seismic codes by 2008, which is expected to cost $10 billion, Richter said. All hospitals must be in "substantial compliance" with the state's stricter seismic safety law by 2030, at an estimated additional cost of $12 billion.

Hurricanes, tornadoes and earthquakes are common enough that no one questions the need for disaster plans to deal with them. But hospital and other health care officials also stay alert to rarer phenomena.

After a tsunami wiped out three Papua New Guinea island villages in July 1998, California officials began to develop disaster plans in case of tidal waves. The state has "started putting signs up along the ocean showing tsunami escape routes," Richter said, adding, "That's another thing our hospitals will have to take into consideration."

History and experience have taught important lessons about what health care professionals can expect when natural disasters strike. Perhaps the most important lesson of all is to expect the unexpected.

SICK AND TIRED

The Great Depression Took a Terrible Toll on Public Health

by Jon Asplund

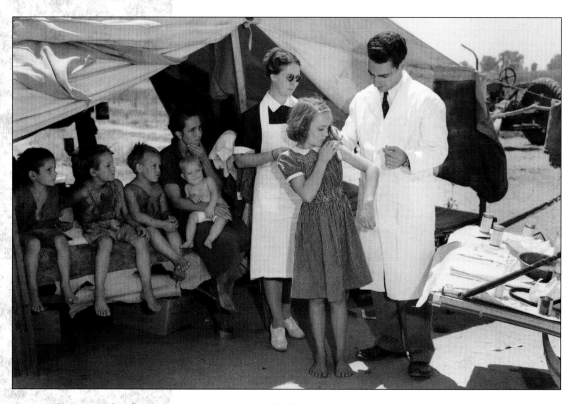

Despite the Roosevelt administration's Depression relief programs, impoverished Americans suffered the long-term effects of malnutrition and lack of medical care. Children in California and other rural regions were immunized against typhoid and smallpox by federally funded physicians who traveled the nation practicing at migrant workers' camps. Source: Corbis-Bettmann

President Franklin D. Roosevelt acknowledged that during the height of the Great Depression he saw "one-third of a nation ill-housed, ill-clad, ill-nourished."

He failed to mention just plain ill.

The decade-long crisis, marked by skyrocketing unemployment, usually is remembered as an economic catastrophe. From the stock market crash of Oct. 29, 1929, until the start of World War II, Americans suffered.

The nation's unemployment rate soared from 3 percent in 1925 to 25 percent in 1933. For those lucky enough to have jobs, wages plummeted. So did prices for goods and services. Some 5,000 banks failed between 1930 and 1933. By 1932, an estimated 25,000 families and more than 200,000 young people were wandering the country, seeking food, shelter and jobs.

Relief came in the form Roosevelt's New Deal programs.

Although projects like dam construction and artists' murals might be remembered most vividly, health care was an important part of New Deal policies.

According to a Depression-era National Health Survey, sponsored by the United States Public Health Service, "every year some 2 million cases of serious illness go entirely without medical treatment," said Florence Kerr, assistant commissioner, Work Projects Administration (WPA), during a 1939 speech. "That is why the WPA maintains and assists clinics in most of our cities. That is why it sends nurses into the homes of the poor. That is why it builds hospitals and provides medical and dental treatment for people who could not receive such treatment otherwise.

"In the first three years of the program [begun in 1933], WPA built over 100 new hospitals and improved 1,422. It has provided technical and clerical workers for city health departments. It has organized and helped conduct maternal and child health clinics in hundreds of communities."

Little Relief

Still, relief efforts often only broke the surface. Consider Martha Gellhorn's November 1934 report on Gaston County, NC. The agent of the Federal Emergency Relief Administration said the county was "a concentration of all evils" and "my idea of a place to go to acquire melancholia."

"The medical setup in this area is nonexistent . . . . Syphilis [is] uncured and unchecked; spread by ignorant people who have no conception of the disease . . . .

"The doctors all talk of malnutrition and fear the present and future effects. Birth control is needed here almost more than in any other area I have ever seen . . . . None of this is surprising; Gaston County has one health office and that's all in the way of public medicine . . . . The private doctors do what they can which isn't much . . . . A generation is being born which will be unfit for any work, unfit to take any place in a decent community."

Similar stories came from relief agent Henry W. Francis, reporting on Logan and Mingo counties in West Virginia. Delbarton, WV, physician R.L. Farley, M.D., told Francis, "Health conditions here are worse than anywhere in the United States . . . . Right now pneumonia is raging throughout these hills. People, lacking clothes but having relief coal or digging it in the hills, heat their hovels to suffocating temperatures. When the fires go out at night the temperature inside the shacks, open as they are, is the same as that outside. Bed clothing is scant and they sleep cold. Children, sleeping on floors, can't help getting pneumonia. I've half a dozen cases to see today."

Care for the Poorest

Urban areas seemed to fare better.

"As for health, the lowest classes are better off," New York City relief agent Wayne W. Parish wrote in 1934. "I am referring to the minority of clients who were always in the poverty classification and who never had permanent homes or jobs. Now they have medical care and go to clinics, and some take advantage of educational facilities which they never had before . . . .

"It is probably a safe conclusion that health conditions are worse among the better class of relief clients because of their inability to use private facilities they formerly enjoyed . . . .

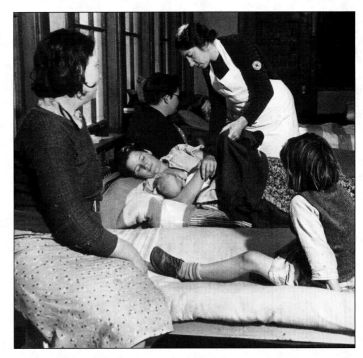

Many urban Americans fared better but still suffered the health effects of poverty. In 1938, patients who could not afford care often were welcome in hospital wards. Source: Corbis-Bettmann

"Mentally, the havoc wreaked among skilled and white collar people cannot be estimated, but it is serious. Many skilled men will never be useful again because of this interlude of worry."

Lingering Effects

America mobilized for war less than a decade later and afterward, during years of prosperity and hope, survivors put the lingering effects of malnutrition and lack of health care behind them. However, there's evidence to suggest the Depression's effect was felt.

In 1940, Brigadier General Lewis B. Hershey, deputy director of the Selective Service System, revealed that "out of a million men examined by Selective Service and about 560,000 excepted by the army, a total of 380,000 have been found unfit for general military service. It has been estimated that perhaps one-third of the rejections were due either directly or indirectly to nutritional deficiencies.

"In terms of men, the army today has been deprived of 150,000 who should be able to do duty as soldiers. This is 15 percent of the total number physically examined by the Selective Service System.

"It is perhaps of little use to speculate on what should have been done by our schools, by parents, by health bodies, or by the government. Probably the Depression years left their marks."

X-RAY VISIONARIES

*A Century of Advances in Medical Imaging Has Led to a New Way
of Seeing and Treating the Human Body*

by Jack Bess

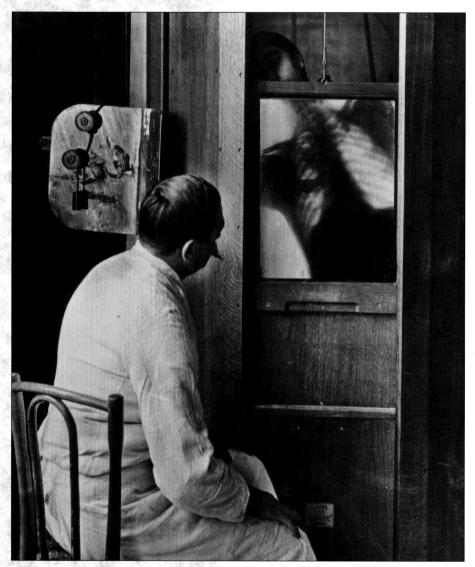

A physician uses a fluoroscopic screen to conduct a radiographic examination of a patient's thorax in 1895. Less than a year later, Wilhelm Roentgen's report on experiments with electromagnetic radiation launched a revolution in how doctors saw and perceived the human body. In the succeeding 100 years, medical imaging has come a long way in what it is capable of showing.

Source: Corbis-Bettmann

In January 1896, seeing was more than believing. It was knowing. Published in January of that year, German physicist Wilhelm Roentgen's report on experiments with the electromagnetic radiation he dubbed "X-rays" inaugurated a new era of medical knowledge and treatment in which machines re-created seemingly miraculous images from inside the human body.

"There were certain things that changed overnight," says Bettyann Holtzmann Kevles, science writer and author of *Naked to the Bone: Origins and Development of Medical Imaging*. "The whole treatment of bullet wounds and fractures changes almost immediately."

Mere months after Roentgen's report was published, the Italian army was X-raying its wounded in field hospitals and the British were following suit in their own imperial campaigns, Kevles says.

Bullet-wound treatment advanced remarkably, compared with the efforts of physicians treating President James Garfield, wounded by an assassin's bullet in 1881. At Garfield's bedside, Alexander Graham Bell used a "sound-induction machine" that would ring when it detected the slug. The experiment failed. Garfield died 80 days after being shot.

The fledgling technology was immediately embraced. This new way of seeing helped lead to a new way of thinking.

The X-ray dovetailed with the "scientific medicine" movement, which helped medicine evolve into a clinical science, Kevles writes: "At the time, doctors were still thinking in terms of idiosyncrasy—the idea that disease is unique to the patient who happens to be peculiarly susceptible to a specific condition. This was the opposite of scientific medicine, where like causes were assumed to produce like symptoms."

Deadly Effects

But while the X-ray brought enormous life-saving benefits, it was also the first technology with a "long, deadly fuse" in that it carried a hidden, delayed risk, Kevles says.

The hazards of prolonged exposure to X-rays became apparent to Thomas Edison. The famed inventor halted his own experiments with X-rays in 1902, after he suffered skin rashes and an assistant gradually lost facial hair, including eyelashes, hair from his scalp and eventually his entire left hand because of radiation poisoning.

Later, scientists would learn that prolonged X-ray exposure can kill.

They learned to take precautions, including placing a leaden screen between the X-ray technician and the patient.

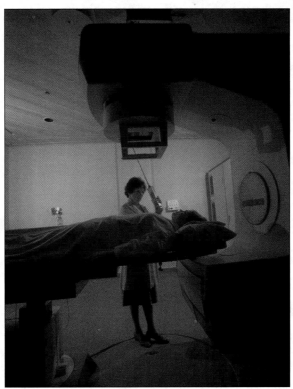

A technician monitors a patient in a magnetic resonance imaging scanner, technology that was introduced in the 1970s. Source: Corbis/Ed Eckstein

Computerized tomography emerged in 1972. CT produces cross-sectional images by passing X-rays through the body. As the X-rays leave, a detector measures and converts them into electrical signals that are converted into numerical data that a computer uses to reconstruct the image.

The CT scanner was developed by Godfrey Hounsfield, an engineer employed by EMI Limited (Electric and Musical Industries) in England, where he researched techniques in image processing and reconstruction.

When Hounsfield received the Nobel Prize in physiology or medicine in 1979 for his work, he shared the honor with Tufts University physics Professor Allan Cormack, who in the 1960s had worked out the mathematics used in measuring X-ray absorption in the body.

Economics of X-rays

The CT scanner was, Kevles says, "the first of the big-ticket body-penetrating cross-sectional imaging machines." The enormous expense of the equipment

prompted states to enact certificate-of-need laws, which required hospitals to prove that they were not duplicating equipment available nearby, Kevles says.

Other landmarks in medical imaging include:

- Magnetic resonance imaging emerged in the late 1970s and was used to image tissue.
- Positron emission tomography, in which images are created by tracing radioactive isotopes injected into the body. The first PET scanner was built in 1976 at Washington University in St. Louis.
- Ultrasound machines, which the Smith-Kline Corp. began to market following successful clinical trials in 1964 at the University of Washington in Seattle, Kevles writes.
- Mammography. While using X-rays to detect breast cancer had been done for years, the procedure was "revolutionized," as Kevles puts it, in 1960 when Robert Egan at the M.D. Anderson Hospital in Houston used high-resolution industrial film in his tests.

Power to the Patient

Imaging technology lets the patient see what the doctor sees, and thereby opens the door to giving patients a role in their own treatment, Kevles says. For example, when the feminist movement of the early 1970s challenged the authority of the male-dominated medical establishment, ultrasound and mammography provided the means by which women could inform themselves, she says.

"Women have learned to read their own mammograms and discuss what [option] is better," Kevles says. "They know what they are looking for. This is part of the generally raised medical knowledge of the layperson . . . . Many physicians I speak to are really very happy to share pictures with a patient. They can say, 'Here is the picture, there is where your problem lies, this is what we can do.' The right attitude can empower the patient and the doctor."

WRITING FROM WITHIN

*Postcards from the Bedside Reveal Our Uneasy
Relationship with Illness*

by Elizabeth Oplatka

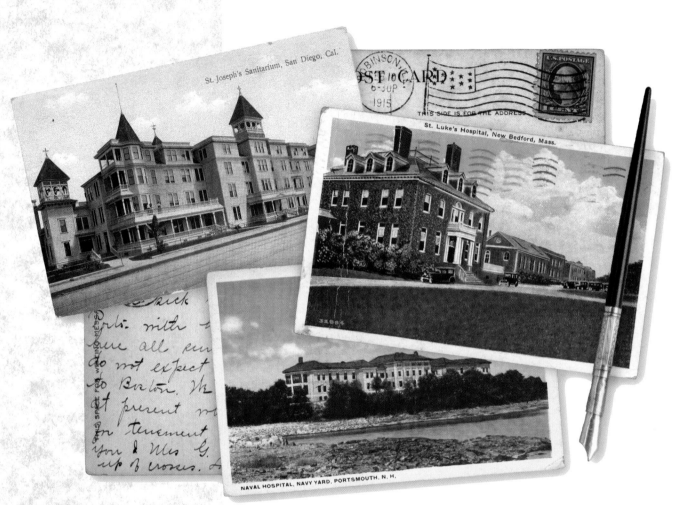

Source: AHA Archives

Historians comb through long-dead national figures' correspondence searching for a mirror on our relationship with history. Researchers at the AHA Resource Center collect postcards written by hospital patients and the loved ones at their bedsides, hoping to reveal the mystery behind our relationship with illness.

Since 1993, the AHA Center for Hospital and Healthcare Administration History has purchased and received donations of nearly 3,000 postcards from collectors. The oldest of the cards dates back to 1905, the most modern was printed in 1984. They range from the resort-like "hand-colored" garden scenes of the Hill House Sanitarium in Martinsville, IN, to the expanse of lawn in front of the Iowa State Hospital for the Insane in Independence. Many contain messages from those seeking a cure.

"The comments are like snapshots of life as a patient," AHA Resource Center Director Eloise Foster says. "They reveal patients' interactions with the environment around them and with the hospitals that delivered their care."

To Chaplain Dick Millspaugh, director of pastoral care at Boone Hospital Center, Columbia, MO, the messages reveal our eternal quest to grasp the human condition.

"What you are trying to do when you read all these cards and letters is exactly what a patient is trying to do in the hospital," Millspaugh says. "You are trying to put meaning on experience. Part of what we're reading is a clue into the human need to find meaning and worth. If I'm sick, does that mean that I am broken from the relationships that usually sustain me? Does this mean that I can no longer count on the people I've always relied on? Am I worthless?"

'Why Haven't You Written?'

In their search for meaning, hospitalized correspondents write home begging for family contact:

"I know you must know I'm here," a man writes in 1908 from his Oklahoma City hospital bed. "Why haven't you written? Please, please let me hear from you."

As seriously ill patients reflect on their lives, they begin to express guilt for neglecting valuable relationships, Millspaugh says. This "life review" raises new regrets. A patient at Burbank Hospital, Fitchburg, MA, who signs her card "Mother," writes in 1913 to her stepdaughter in South Eliot, ME. The woman, who says that she "can just now sit up in bed," appears racked with guilt for failing to write:

"My precious little girl, just thinking how I neglected you in writing to you, hope you will forgive one for

doing so. I promise I want to write you again and again, my loving stepdaughter. I love you and never mean to neglect you like this, I must try and do better."

Families likely found some messages home more disturbing than others. An author who signs himself "M" writes in 1908 on a postcard picturing the Danvers, MA, Hospital for the Insane:

"Dear Mother, This card will tell you where I am and what I'm doing. As usual have been here near two months. Like very well. Hope you are feeling better."

Notes from patients' bedsides stress details of their loved ones' illnesses and prospects for the future. Millspaugh says that many of the writers are preparing distant relatives for the inevitable:

"Dear brother . . . Uncle Lamb is awful bad sick with asthma," John W. Shire writes W.D. Walker from Hill House Sanitarium, Martinsville, IN, in February 1915, ". . . liable to drop off at any time."

"By preparing their families, loved ones at the bedside are helping the family get in touch with mortality and begin grieving," Millspaugh says. "They are calling on the relationships within their community—mother, son, brother, sister, pastor—to rally around."

The attentive daughter of an elderly hospitalized woman empathizes with another elderly patient who has no one at her bedside:

"There is an 80 year old woman and a 57 year old woman in the room with mama," the writer identified as "Thelda" writes from Elizabeth Hospital, Prairie Grove, AR, in 1956. "The 80 yr. old is the mother of 17 children and no one comes to see her. I comb her hair when I comb Mama's."

"As our sensitivity grows, our acts of kindness take on extraordinary meaning and to the patient, they feel just wonderful," Millspaugh says. "The recipients of such kindness feel like they're being seen and understood."

Years ago, hospitals did not have phones at the bedside. Cards and letters were the primary source of communication. Millspaugh wonders whether modern correspondence would reflect historical emotions.

"Since most people now talk on the phone, we might never know whether the feelings expressed in these letters are limited by their moment in history," Millspaugh says. "As a chaplain, I wonder whether the experience of my patients is any different."

The AHA Resource Center collects hospital postcards. To donate or view the collection, you may contact the center at (312) 422-2000.

RESTORATION WORK

*Helping WW II Amputees Transformed VA into a Leader
in Medical Research*

by Chris Larson

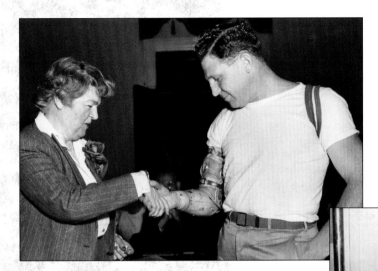

*U.S. Rep. Edith Nourse Rogers of Massachusetts gets an
enthusiastic handshake from Pfc. Leo Qualiotto (left)
after a number of veterans who lost limbs in World War
II appeared before the House Veterans Affairs
Committee in April 1947. The veterans demonstrated
various experimental prostheses being developed by the
Veterans Administration. Qualiotto lost his arm at
Normandy.   Source: Corbis-Bettmann*

*Marine Pvt. Ralph J. Theis (right), who lost both feet on
Guadalcanal is attended by a staff member at Oak Knoll
Naval Hospital, San Francisco.   Source: Corbis-Bettmann*

As World War II neared its end, the health care
system was dealing with the many amputee soldiers who required rehabilitation.

Yet prosthetic devices were still crude. A century
after the Civil War first created a large population of
amputees, a coordinated effort into research and development had never materialized.

That changed after World War II, as the Veterans
Administration (now the Department of Veterans Affairs)
launched joint research projects to advance the field of
prosthetics. It was among the first major VA research projects, and paved the way for many of the contributions the
VA has made to American health care.

Little research was conducted at early VA hospitals,
records show. And though some research was conducted
in the decade after World War II, research wasn't an official part of the VA's mission until 1958. That year, a

Senate committee report called for an "accelerated program" of VA research to cut costs and improve treatment
so veterans could "return to normal living."

Many American companies made prostheses prior to
World War II, but there was no government-sponsored
research effort to advance the field, said Dudley
Childress, director of the Prosthetics Research Lab at
Northwestern University medical school.

In 1945, the surgeon general held a meeting of physicians and engineers in Chicago to study how to treat the
many amputee veterans who soon would return home.

"Out of that meeting came the concept of a federally
assisted program to get things moving," Childress said.

The first grants, which funded the VA and other research projects, were awarded in 1946, Childress said. The grants led to advances in hydraulic knee mechanisms and artificial feet. Refinements also were made to the "socket," the point of contact between the body and prosthesis.

Meanwhile, VA-funded projects at various universities were studying the functions of the hands and the mechanics of walking. Other researchers worked to refine amputation techniques.

Many VA medical advances have been related to the needs of the military. Post-traumatic stress disorder— once known as shellshock—has received much attention from VA researchers.

Many of the VA's treatment findings have been applied successfully to rape victims and other abuse patients, said Don Mickey, director of the VA Research Communications Service.

Invisible Wounds
Similarly, the VA has conducted much research into schizophrenia, Mickey said, because the disease often first occurs in patients in their early 20s—the most common age of military recruits. The VA operates schizophrenia treatment centers nationwide.

Other advances have come in fields not specific to veterans. The cardiac pacemaker, for example, was developed at a VA hospital in Buffalo, NY. Much of the early research into tuberculosis was performed by the VA "simply because many veterans hospitals were dedicated to long-term care for TB patients," Mickey said. "The physicians who cared for these patients started protocols to find new treatments for them."

Other VA advances include the vaccine for hepatitis B, and the first liver and kidney transplants, according to VA documents. Two VA scientists, Rosalyn Yalow and

Andrew Schally, shared the 1977 Nobel Prize for their work in radioisotopes and brain hormones, respectively.

Many discoveries have been made because the VA's chief medical director, Paul B. Magnuson, M.D., in the 1940s believed that affiliations between medical schools and VA medical centers would assist research. Today, each of the nearly 100 VA medical centers that perform research is affiliated with a school, Mickey said.

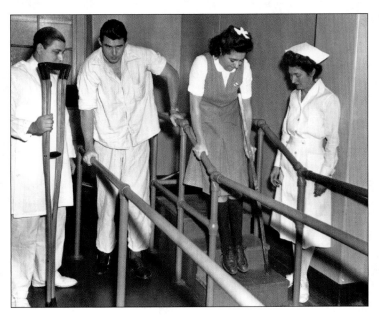

Members of the medical staff at a Veterans Administration Hospital in New York City watch as a Marine Corps veteran and a former member of the Women's Army Corps practice rehabilitation exercises in December 1944. Both veterans were wounded in World War II. The Veterans Administration got involved in prosthetic research because of the large numbers of amputees returning home from the war and the crude artificial limbs then available. Source: Corbis-Bettmann

Study Needed
Research continues at the VA. Illnesses among Gulf War veterans is a major area of interest, Mickey said. Prosthetics are still heavily studied, with recent advances in the computer-aided design and manufacturing of prosthetic devices. The VA also is active in studies of improved wound treatments and is a leader in the field of spinal-cord regeneration and injury treatment. VA researchers also investigate fields not related to combat. The department is active in research into tuberculosis and AIDS. The aging veteran population allows the VA to research various effects and diseases of old age, Mickey said.

In percentage terms, the VA doesn't spend much money on research.

Less than 2 percent of the VA's total medical expenditures for 1998 is slated for research. But add that $272 million to the National Institutes of Health and the National Science Foundation grants awarded VA researchers and $650 million will be spent by the VA on medical research in 1998.

Although its primary mission is to serve veterans, VA research ultimately assists all patients. "VA research doesn't just help veterans," Mickey said. "It helps anyone who needs those findings. There are no diseases or medical problems that are unique to veterans."

SET FREE

Once Considered Humane, the Wholesale Release of Mentally Ill Patients Is Now under Scrutiny

by Chris Larson

This was supposed to be a good thing. Deinstitutionalization—releasing patients from mental hospitals and integrating them back into society—started in the 1950s. Experts could see that the poor and abusive conditions at crowded, understaffed hospitals were actually making the conditions of many patients worse. With the development of new medications, experts began to believe that many patients would be better served outside of mental hospitals.

"There was nothing wrong with the concept," said E. Fuller Torrey, M.D., executive director of the Stanley Foundation research programs. "The concept was perfectly sound and humane. The problem was the execution, which was basically emptying out the hospitals without making sure that the people got the medication they needed to remain relatively symptom-free."

Deinstitutionalization has dramatically lowered the number of mentally ill hospital patients: the mental hospital population peaked at more than 550,000 in the mid-1950s, statistics show; today, there are around 70,000 patients in U.S. mental hospitals.

Many former patients have led productive lives outside of hospitals. Yet large numbers have not received the continued treatment their conditions require. Many end up homeless, in jail, or otherwise a burden on society.

The deinstitutionalization movement began slowly as new drugs became available. In New York, for example, the number of hospitalized mentally ill patients dropped

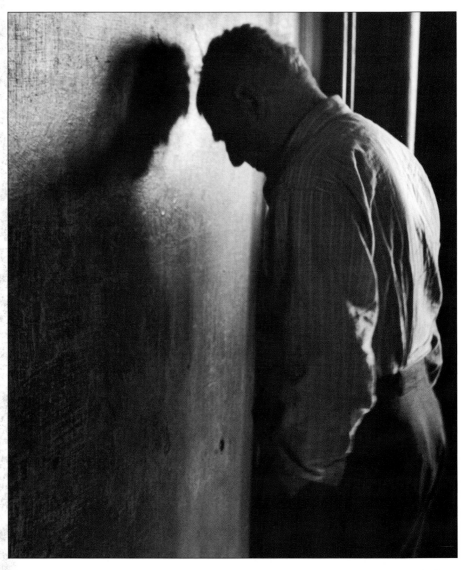

Poor conditions at mental hospitals in the 1950s led experts to embrace a system of "deinstitutionalization," which was intended to integrate patients back into society. Many patients, like the man above in an Ohio hospital in 1946, spent hours alone with nothing to occupy their time because there were not enough staff members to supervise activities.

Source: Corbis/Jerry Cooke

from 93,000 in 1955 to 89,000 in 1959, records show. Meanwhile, a congressional commission in 1955 began to study the state of American mental health care.

One of its conclusions—that a network of community services was needed to help patients readjust—led to the

1963 passage of the Community Mental Health Centers Act. The law created federally funded community centers offering such services as job counseling and outpatient psychiatric care.

But there weren't enough centers, and many were underfunded.

"It could have been a much more successful process had the [support] infrastructure been built more quickly and had there been better funding," said Irma J. Bland, M.D., chair of the AHA's Section for Psychiatric and Substance Abuse Services and regional medical director for the Louisiana Office of Mental Health.

An Issue of Civil Rights

Court decisions in the late 1960s and 1970s sped up the process, as hospitalization of mentally ill patients became a civil rights issue. "Laws were changed in most of the states, making it much easier to get people out, very difficult to get them back in, and almost impossible to treat involuntarily," Torrey said.

Another major problem, Torrey added, is the nature of mental illness itself. "About half of the people we were releasing didn't think there was anything wrong with them, because of their brain disease," he said. "There's no way these people were going to take their medication."

Recent studies found that more state hospital beds were lost in the 1980s and '90s than in the '60s and '70s, even as social service budgets were being cut.

"What we saw in the 1980s, and even today, is more homeless people with severe mental illnesses, and a shift toward jails and prisons," said Andrew Sperling, director of public policy at the National Alliance for the Mentally Ill (NAMI).

Conservative estimates are that 150,000 of the nation's 500,000 homeless are mentally ill, as are another 150,000 of the 1.5 million jail and prison inmates. "We also estimate that there are about a thousand murders committed annually [out of a total of 24,000] by seriously mentally ill people who are not on medication," Torrey added.

About 40 percent of the unhospitalized mentally ill are untreated on any given day, according to the National Institute of Mental Health.

"NAMI largely believes that deinstitutionalization failed," Sperling said. "Not because we believe we ought to reopen large state hospitals, but because the community support and services never really came about."

That remains a major concern. "Building the infrastructure of support, and having the financial resources to maintain that infrastructure adequately, is the primary issue," Bland said.

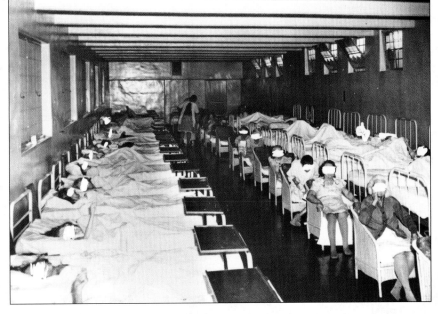

Many patients in a crowded ward for aged women at a California state mental hospital in 1949 were forced to sleep on chairs or on cushions placed on floors. Experts say many deinstitutionalized patients ended up homeless or in jail because governments did not adequately fund community mental health centers where patients could receive counseling and drug supervision. But new medications are raising hopes that patients can lead relatively normal lives outside hospitals.

Source: Corbis-Bettmann

"Getting adequate moneys to provide those services continues to be an extreme challenge."

But there is hope. "Over the past decade, medications have gotten much, much better," Bland said. "Medications today are much more effective at helping people with severe illnesses come out of hospitals and into communities."

"Most of these people don't need to be in a hospital. They need to be on their medication," Torrey said. "We have to look at the medication effort. That involves involuntary treatment, which is politically incorrect to talk about, but that is the reality."

Bland and many experts remain optimistic. "We're hopeful because, conceptually, we know what's necessary, and we know the kinds of successes that patients can have," Bland said.

AGE OF ENLIGHTENMENT

How Compassion and Professionalism Replaced the Fear of AIDS

by Jack Bess

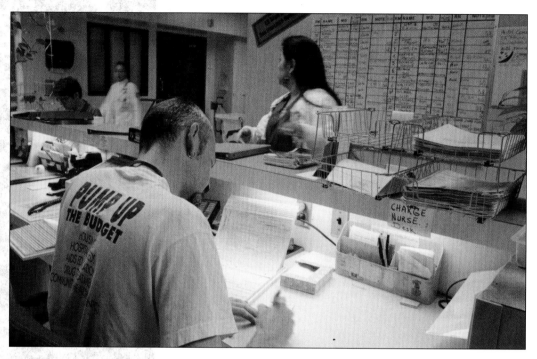

San Francisco General Hospital launched the nation's first AIDS unit (shown above in 1995 photo), creating a seamless support network for the patient, inside and outside the hospital. Patients' loved ones held Sunday brunches on the unit and were included in discussions about treatment. In the early years of the epidemic, patients encountered bigotry and fear from the staffs at many hospitals. But when hospitals started to establish units dedicated to AIDS, nurses were given a strong voice in the design and policy and helped change attitudes about AIDS patients hospitalwide.

Source: San Francisco General Hospital

At a time when some hospitalized AIDS patients complained of society's bigotry and isolation, Gloria Taylor decided she wanted to erase the distance between care-giver and patient.

Taylor landed a job as a nurse at St. Clare's Hospital and Health Center in New York City in 1985, just as the hospital was forming a special unit dedicated to AIDS patients. It was as if her sense of justice and her professional calling merged.

Taylor had heard patients' stories about nurses who didn't check on them frequently enough and meal trays left outside hospital room doors.

"Someone I loved very dearly had died from AIDS," said Taylor, now the hospital's nursing director. "I always thought he deserved better. I thought everybody else deserved better."

Such intense commitment helped create a new mode of nursing in hospitals' dedicated AIDS units. Not only did nurses have a stronger voice in the design and policy of these units, they also helped change attitudes about AIDS patients hospitalwide.

When Fear Reigned

In the early 1980s, when mystery surrounded the issue of how AIDS was transmitted, some health care workers struggled with the same fears about AIDS patients that were felt in society at-large.

"People seemed to die very rapidly of the disease once it was identified," said Gayling Gee, formerly a nurse at San Francisco General Hospital's AIDS clinic and now associate administrator of the hospital's community health network. "It would make [hospital staff] very concerned about their personal safety because they knew that the disease was infectious."

The fear was such that some medical personnel "would put on all the protective clothing just for a noninvasive procedure like an electrocardiogram," said Karen Coleman, nurse manager at Illinois Masonic Medical Center in Chicago.

When Illinois Masonic created an AIDS unit in 1985, "we could not get nurses to float into this unit, and the nursing administration supported that [decision]," Coleman said.

San Francisco General Hospital led the way for other institutions by launching the nation's first AIDS unit in 1983.

Clinical nurse specialist Cliff Morrison spearheaded the effort to create a seamless network of support for the patient, inside and outside the hospital.

Psychiatric and social services were available at the unit, and social workers kept in touch with discharged patients. Patients' loved ones held Sunday brunches on the unit and were included in discussions about treatment. Nurses spent more time with fewer patients than in a conventional hospital setting.

"I've been in nursing 35 years, and when I came [to the Illinois Masonic unit] 10 years ago, it reinforced and renewed my reasons for wanting to be a nurse," Coleman said. "I felt so needed."

Team Effort
This practice environment appealed to many nurses, said Linda Aiken, director of the Center for Health Services and Policy Research at the University of Pennsylvania's School of Nursing.

Hospitals "would turn these units over to nurses" who designed them to reflect the type of care that "nurses always wanted. There were interdisciplinary teams—doctors, nurses, health professionals, occupational therapists—all working together," Aiken said.

Hospital officials who had been "afraid there would not be enough nurses for AIDS care," now found themselves with waiting lists of nurses wanting to work in the units, Aiken said. "The environment was attractive and consistent with their beliefs about what nursing was."

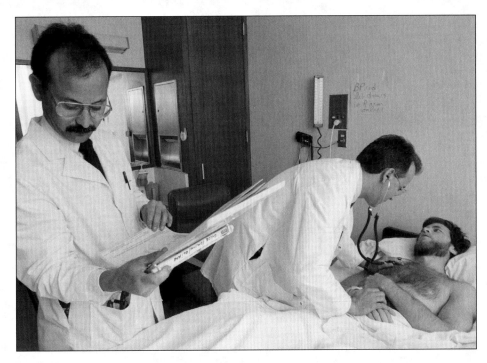

Physicians check on a person with AIDS in a Seattle hospital in 1987.

Source: Corbis/Roger Ressmeyer

At St. Clare's, nurses helped develop protocols and write a training manual for care-givers—covering everything from nutrition to spirituality—that is still used as a teaching tool, Taylor said.

And at Illinois Masonic, nurses successfully pushed for a change in the "very restrained" visiting-hours policy, so loved ones could stay overnight in the AIDS unit, Coleman said.

Experience in the AIDS unit enabled nurses to become teachers to the rest of hospital staff, educating them about the disease and showing that "all the protective clothing" wasn't necessary to prevent transmission of the virus, Coleman said.

Male Nurses' Role
The AIDS epidemic "transformed" the role of male nurses, Aiken said. Traditionally, there was a "certain discomfort" with male nurses in clinical roles, so they would go into administrative roles, she said. But the AIDS crisis increased the number of male nurses and "created a more legitimate clinical role" for them, she said.

St. Clare's saw a surge of male nurses, some of them retired or moonlighting police officers and firefighters who requested assignment at the AIDS unit, Taylor said.

Working at the unit was one of the most important experiences of her life, Taylor said.

"It took this horrible, horrible thing for us to realize how fragile we are and how much we have in common with other people," she said.

WHERE MEDICINE MET CIVIL RIGHTS

Health Care Professionals Were Among the First to Fight for Disabled Americans

by Jack Bess

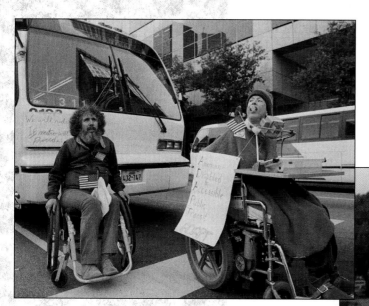

Disabled Americans' protests (left) helped lead to the passage of the Americans with Disabilities Act (ADA) in 1990. Members of Accessible Public Transportation blocked Houston city buses demanding buses with wheelchair lifts.

Source: Corbis-Bettmann/UPI

President George Bush signs the ADA during a ceremony on the South Lawn of the White House (right). Disability rights activists the Rev. Harold Wilke (rear left); Evan Kemp, chairman of the Equal Opportunity Employment Commission (front left); Sandra Parrino, chair of the National Council on Disability (right rear); and Justin Dart, chairman of the President's Council on Disabilities attended the signing.

Source: AP/Wide World Photo

What's the difference between a person with a disability and a person without a disability? Sometimes it's a matter of perspective.

In 1971, Jann Dragovich crossed the border between two states of mind when she met a 21-year-old man who had lost a leg to cancer and wore a prosthetic limb.

"I couldn't believe he was married," she recalls. "I thought nothing in the world could be worse and that I'd rather be dead before someone takes apart my body."

Not long afterward, Dragovich lost one of her legs in a motorcycle accident. Returning to school, she studied rehabilitation counseling and joined a growing movement of people with disabilities working to secure their civil rights. Today she is the executive director of the Center for Disability and Elder Law in Chicago, founded in 1983 to provide free legal services to disabled and senior citizens.

Different World
The center represents an immeasurable advance from the reality disabled people faced only a few decades ago.

"From the 1920s to the 1970s, the theme of separation predominated in all of the government's social welfare programs," writes Edward D. Berkowitz in his book *Disabled Policy: America's Programs for the Handicapped.*

"Income-maintenance programs asked the handicapped to remove themselves from the labor force in order to receive government aid," Berkowitz writes.

Drawing borders—physical and social—between people with disabilities and the rest of society also was practiced in health care, says Henry Betts, M.D., foundation chairman of the Rehabilitation Institute of Chicago, where he went to work in 1963 as a physician and proved himself a passionate advocate of disabled Americans' rights.

"Where I interned [in the 1950s], people with spinal cord injuries were put in boxes with sawdust in the bottom of them that looked like coffins," Betts says. "It was very handy for the incontinent. You could just shovel away the sawdust."

Another Civil-Rights Movement

People with disabilities were treated in ways that recalled the segregated South of Betts' childhood. In one institution, the physical therapy room was relegated to the basement near the heating pipes and boiler room. And when Betts took a residency in California, he saw a rehabilitation area created by blocking off an abandoned corridor.

Such treatment, and the basic idea that people with disabilities would agree to stay out of sight in exchange for government assistance, would begin to be re-examined and rejected in the 1960s, when the budding disability-rights movement drew energy and inspiration from other civil-rights struggles and anti-war protests.

A key figure in this movement was Judy Heumann, now an officer in the U.S. Department of Education. A post-polio syndrome survivor who uses a wheelchair, Heumann was turned down in 1970 when she applied for a teaching license at the New York City Public Schools, which cited concern for the safety of her students. She filed a discrimination suit against the board in federal court, and the irony of her situation, Berkowitz notes, was caught by a *New York Daily News* headline: "You Can Be President, Not Teacher, with Polio."

In 1972, other disabled activists founded the Berkeley, CA, Center for Independent Living. Setting an example

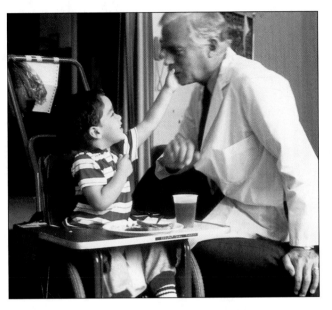

Henry Betts, M.D., foundation chairman of the Rehabilitation Institute of Chicago, said he learned early in his career that caring for disabled patients largely was a matter of advocating for their civil rights.

Source: Rehabilitation Institute of Chicago

eventually replicated in other cities, the center provided to people with disabilities services "that the handicapped can control on their own terms, and it is dedicated to independence and the transcendence of other institutions," Berkowitz writes.

Where Medicine Meets Civil Rights

Health care institutions still play a critical role in educating the rest of society, Betts says. The Rehabilitation Institute "delved very, very deeply into the community," bringing business people onto its board and putting them at the heart of policy discussions. Such inclusion works, and the board sometimes comes up with its own initiatives, such as its annual cash award to someone who works to improve the quality of life for disabled citizens. "This is not a bunch of do-gooders or philosophers," Betts says. "These are business people. It gives you an idea of how deeply felt this goal [of equality] is," he says.

The eloquence of disabled activists, plus a new awareness in society at-large, led the way for the passage of the landmark Americans with Disabilities Act (ADA) in 1990. A comprehensive law that prohibits discrimination and sets accessibility standards for new construction and existing buildings, the ADA is "the beacon for the whole world to look at," Betts says. But a law is not the whole solution, he adds. As awareness grows, so does the recognition of the need for new services.

In 1990, two female physicians at the Rehabilitation Institute realized that disabled women weren't getting routine breast and pelvic exams or being treated for sexually transmitted diseases, says Judy Panko Reis, administrative director of the Institute's Health Resource Center for Women with Disabilities, founded in 1991. Some male doctors thought disabled women were not having sex and that it would be "pathological" for such women to want to bear children, she says.

"We're trying to demythologize disability," she says. "If people are going to insist that disability is an abnormality, people are going to feel that way about themselves."

Early Birth, Early Death

Until the Mid-20th Century, Medical Science Could Do Very Little for Premature Babies

by Gloria Shur Bilchik

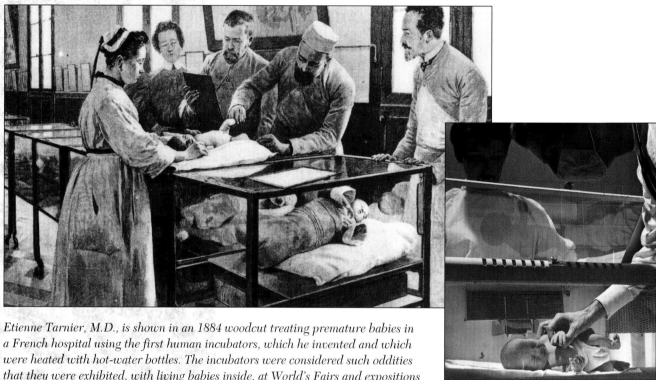

Etienne Tarnier, M.D., is shown in an 1884 woodcut treating premature babies in a French hospital using the first human incubators, which he invented and which were heated with hot-water bottles. The incubators were considered such oddities that they were exhibited, with living babies inside, at World's Fairs and expositions until the 1930s. It wasn't until the middle of this century that major technological and medical advances were made in treating premature babies. At right, a doctor examines a tiny infant in a New York City hospital incubator in 1958.

Sources: Corbis-Bettmann (top), Corbis/Jerry Cooke (right)

Patrick Bouvier Kennedy, perhaps the most famous premature baby of the 20th century, was born— too soon and too small—on Aug. 7, 1963. Five weeks early, he was delivered by emergency C-section at Otis Air Force Base Hospital in Barnstable, MA, after his mother, Jacqueline, was rushed by helicopter from the Kennedy compound in Hyannis. He weighed 4 pounds, 1 ounce.

Like most premature infants of the early 1960s, his chances of survival were slim. His doctors called every colleague they knew, seeking advice. They placed Patrick in a hyperbaric chamber in hope of overcoming the respiratory distress (then known as hyaline membrane disease) caused by his immature lungs. But three days later, he died.

As the son of the president, Patrick Kennedy drew worldwide attention to the problems of caring for premature infants. "The Kennedy story was a big turning point," says Philip Sunshine, M.D., professor of pediatrics at Stanford University, Palo Alto, CA. "After that, federal research money for neonatal care became much easier to get."

That development was long overdue. Until the French Revolution of 1789, infants were not considered human beings and had no rights. And until the late 19th century, doctors generally considered babies born before the expected nine-month gestation period to be incomplete fetal material. In the medical parlance of the day, they were called "weaklings" and their deaths were regarded as nature taking care of itself.

A Matter of Patriotism

The first major shift in attitude came after the Franco-Prussian War of 1870. The conflict decimated a generation of young Frenchmen, creating a deep post-war decline in the birth rate. With its birth rate half that of Germany, France feared for its ability to fight in a future war.

"That's when decreasing the infant mortality rate became a matter of patriotism among French physicians," says William Silverman, M.D., author of *Where's the Evidence?* a collection of essays on the history and social impact of neonatal care.

In 1891, Frenchman Etienne Tarnier, M.D., invented the first human incubator. It was a primitive, double-chambered affair heated by hot-water bottles. "It was considered an oddity—so curious that it was exhibited, with living babies inside, at World's Fairs and expositions in 'Incubator Shows' until the 1930s," Silverman says. "They were not in scientific exhibits, but in the freak shows."

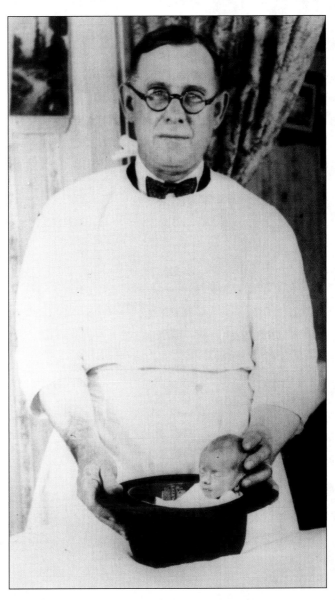

Chicago physician A.H. Farley, M.D., cradles a premature baby in a hat in 1931. The infant weighed only 24 ounces at birth but was expected to survive. Source: Corbis-Bettmann

ventilation by measuring blood oxygenation using only small amounts of drawn blood.

Still, when Patrick Kennedy was born, the state of the art was quite crude, says L. Joseph Butterfield, chairman emeritus of the Department of Perinatology at Children's Hospital, Denver. "We really didn't have a lot to offer. Mechanical ventilation was not a widespread practice. Mostly, we kept babies warm, paid a lot of attention to feeding them, and isolated them—even from their mothers—in hopes of warding off infections." Butterfield opened a newborn center at Children's in 1965. The center's policy of eliminating restrictive visiting hours and allowing "mothering in" set a new standard for nurturing contact.

In the 1970s, neonatology emerged as a pediatric sub-specialty. Physicians began using a technique called continuous positive airway pressure to keep infants' lungs inflated, and researchers continued to

Specialized care for preemies in the U.S. began in the 1940s, when a few hospitals set up "premature-infant stations." By the late 1950s, many hospitals had established the premature nurseries that eventually evolved into today's highly sophisticated neonatal intensive care units.

Evolution of Care

The picture changed dramatically in 1961, when researchers, led by Mildred Stahlman, M.D., of Vanderbilt University, Nashville, TN, figured out how to get air into premature tiny lungs by using a "baby-bird" ventilator. At the same time, new microchemistry techniques enabled physicians to monitor the effectiveness of

refine an artificial placenta (now known as ECMO and widely used). More recently, researchers developed artificial surfactant to replace the soap-like, oxygen-absorbing substance lacking in premature infants' lungs. "This was the previously missing link in respiratory distress syndrome," Butterfield says.

"Until the 1980s, babies born before 28 weeks gestation and weighing under 1,000 grams [about 2 pounds, 9 ounces] had a mortality rate of 80 to 90 percent," Sunshine says. "Now, the viability limit is down to about 24 weeks, and if we can get even the tiniest babies to reach 1,000 grams, they generally survive. We've come a long, long way."

EAT AND BE HEALTHY

Evolution of Hospital Food Reflects Dual Goals of Comfort and Healing

by Gloria Shur Bilchik

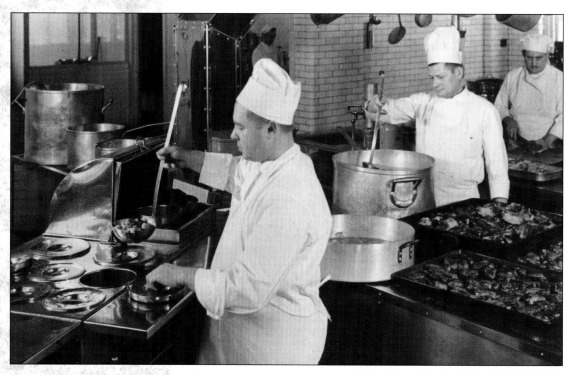

There were never too many cooks to stir the pots in a busy kitchen like this one at Henry Ford Hospital in Detroit in 1930. Henry Ford had strong beliefs about food and nutrition and set aside part of his nearby farm to raise produce for his namesake hospital. His dairy also supplied the hospital with milk, cream and butter. Florence Nightingale made the connection between food and healing during the Crimean War, and science later confirmed her theories, helping to give rise to the dietary sciences.

Photo courtesy of the Henry Ford Health System Archives, Detroit.

Mush and molasses for breakfast and lunch, and perhaps a pint of beer with supper. Hospital patients in the late 1700s were expected to convalesce on a daily diet that was extremely bland, excruciatingly monotonous by modern standards, and only accidentally related to their nutritional needs.

It wasn't until the mid-1850s that the menu began to change. And the catalyst was none other than Florence Nightingale, who enlisted the services of Alexis Soyer, a world-famous chef, to organize diet kitchens in military hospitals during the Crimean War.

From that experience, Nightingale concluded that food made a difference in the patient's recovery. Widely published and accepted, her observations had a permanent influence in medical care.

Later in the 19th century, science began to confirm the connection between food and health. In addition, Americans were acquiring a taste for better food, and cooking schools gained popularity. Sara Tyson Rorer, who operated one of the first, the Philadelphia Cooking School, is widely credited as America's original dietitian.

By the end of the 19th century, nurses' training included cooking classes. At Lowell General Hospital in Massachusetts, for example, nursing students studied under Fanny Farmer, author of the historic *Boston Cook Book*.

By the early 1900s, the field then known as "dietotherapy" was on the rise. In 1917, it gained professional status and a new name with the formation of the American Dietetic Association. Physicians' orders began to include diets tied to specific illnesses. "Dietists" were expected to prepare and serve them.

During this same era, Henry Ford founded his namesake hospital in Detroit, instituting policies that reflected his strong personal beliefs about food and nutrition. Ford set aside a portion of his farm at nearby Dearborn to furnish the hospital with fresh fruits and vegetables. He also established a dairy that supplied milk, cream and butter.

But Is It Good for You?

Through the first half of this century, the standard hospital diet included selections that mimicked home cooking trends of the times. "Bacon, eggs and sausage were typical breakfast choices," says Marilyn Swanson, professor of nutrition at South Dakota State University. "A good person to hire for your dietary department was someone who was a good cook. It didn't matter if they knew anything at all about grams of fat or salt, as long as they could make it look and taste good."

Efficiency was not a priority until very recently. "We had a do-it-yourself mentality," says Jacques Bloch, who served as the first president of the American Society of Hospital Food Service Administrators. At Johns Hopkins Hospital in Baltimore, where Bloch worked in the 1950s, milk was purchased in bulk, then pasteurized and bottled in the hospital's own facilities. Bloch's staff bought sides of beef and lamb and did their own meat cutting. Marilyn

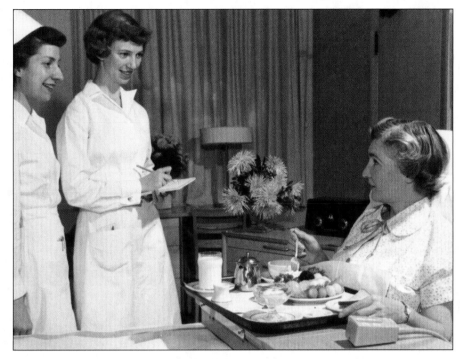

Nurses at Henry Ford Hospital in the 1950s check on a patient to make sure her meal is as good tasting as it is nutritional. As the number of inpatient days drops, hospitals today are experimenting with ways to satisfy patients' palates and to do so as efficiently as possible.   Photo courtesy of the Henry Ford Health System Archives, Detroit.

Swanson recalls visiting a hospital in Idaho in the 1970s, where the cook made noodles from scratch.

The eternal struggle, though, has always been to please patients' palates. As competition among hospitals grew, especially after World War II, patients' menu choices expanded exponentially. (Some hospitals even included matches on the meal tray, so patients could smoke after their meals.) In the 1960s and even into the 1980s, many hospitals hired restaurant or hotel chefs to upgrade quality.

"Some went to silly extremes," says Ellen Luros-Purdy, president of Computrition, of Los Angeles. "I remember looking at one hospital's menu and not being able to pronounce the names of many selections. And some of the menu items, while fancy and elegant-sounding, were so elaborately prepared and so rich that they made no sense for a convalescing patient."

Today, food-industry research reveals that patients stay in hospitals, on average, only long enough to eat 2.5 meals. In fact, many patients are discharged as soon as they can eat a regular meal. As a result, hospitals are reducing menu choices and even moving toward airline-style food service. A few are experimenting with a room-service approach.

Some things, however, remain the same. "No matter what the choices, patients tend to select traditional foods, like macaroni and cheese, mashed potatoes, tomato soup and meatloaf," says Luros-Purdy. "People who are sick want comfort in their foods, too. It looks like we're going back to the old home cooking tradition. Hospital food is coming full circle."

TOOLS OF THE TRADE

*From Stone Age to Present, Instruments Have
Defined and Refined Surgery*

by Gloria Shur Bilchik

Surgical tools from the 17th century bear ornate designs, evidence of doctors' pride of ownership. In the 1930s and 1940s, ownership of instruments began to shift from surgeons to hospitals and clinics. A lithograph from the mid-19th century (inset) reflects how increasingly ambitious surgical techniques led to more complex instruments. In the latter half of the 1800s, surgical instruments became smaller and more delicate as the science of anesthesia shifted the focus of surgery away from amputation and toward preserving limbs and organs. Antiseptic and aseptic techniques revolutionized operating rooms in the late 1800s. Smooth instruments that could withstand high heat and could be disassembled quickly to be sterilized replaced instruments with carved ivory and wooden handles and other hard-to-sterilize parts. Technology has advanced with breathtaking speed in this century, rendering some state-of-the-art instruments obsolete almost as soon as they're introduced, while other standbys continue to be used.

Source: Corbis-Bettmann

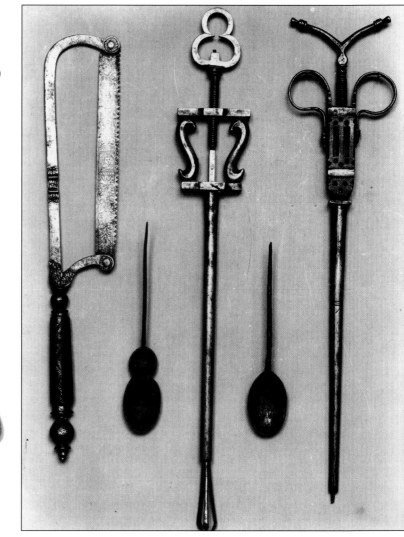

I n the early 1600s in England, obstetrical forceps were a closely guarded trade secret. Literally kept under wraps by their inventors, the Chamberlain brothers, the forceps were used as a last resort in difficult deliveries. They horrified patients, but revolutionized childbirth. And over hundreds of years, through many refinements, they have endured, emblematic of the role instruments have played in advancing medical care, particularly in surgery.

"The practice of surgery—the art, craft and more recently the science—of working with the hands, has always been defined by its tools," says Ira M. Rutkow,

M.D., author of *Surgery, An Illustrated History*. "From the crude flint instruments of Stone Age trephines [used for boring holes in the skull], to the bronze instruments of Egyptian and Roman surgeons, to the increasingly complex surgical instruments developed in the latter half of the 19th century, a better instrument usually led to a better surgical result. Progress in surgical instrumentation and surgical technique went hand in hand."

Fitting the Times

Surgical instruments often have reflected special, ephemeral needs of the times. Joseph O'Dwyer was revered as a hero for American children when he invented an intubation device for diphtheria patients in the mid-1880s. But by the 1890s, when the disease was virtually eradicated by antitoxins and immunizations, O'Dwyer had become a forgotten man.

Another short-lived instrument was invented by Army surgeon Joseph Howland Bill, who served in New Mexico during the U.S. Army's late-19th century campaigns against Native American tribes. In 1876, Bill developed a special forceps for extracting arrowheads from wounds. "It was a quintessential American instrument," says James Edmunson, M.D., author of *American Surgical Instruments, A History of Their Manufacture*. "Gen. George A. Custer and the 7th Cavalry might have used a few of these later that summer."

But some instruments have had impressive staying power. A forceps introduced in the early 1900s by George Crile, M.D., a founding father of the Cleveland Clinic, is still widely used. Similarly, today's surgeons continue to expect to find Metzenbaum scissors, named for their 1920s-era inventor, in the standard surgical setup.

Progress toward Preserving

Until the mid-1840s, most surgical instruments were large, heavy items that reflected the demands of the typically heroic procedures of the day, such as amputations. Between 1840 and 1890, the tools became smaller and more delicate as conservative surgery, assisted by the new science of anesthesia, shifted attention toward preservation of limbs and organs.

The biggest change in instrument design took place in the late 1800s, when antiseptic and aseptic surgical techniques became the norm. Gone was the sword-like amputation knife, as were the carved ivory and wood handles that decorated earlier instruments. Newly instituted sterilization proce-

dures called for smooth instruments that could withstand high heat and that could be disassembled quickly to expose germ-harboring joints and recesses. Also banished were leather cases, lined with silk or velvet, replaced by canvas bags that could be sterilized along with everything else.

Before surgical instrument companies emerged, craftsman, often in the silversmithing, cutlery or blacksmithing trades, executed surgeons' ideas for enhancements. Surgeons traditionally owned their own instruments, often customized to their own preferences. In fact, they were among physicians' most prized possessions. Having invested large amounts of money in the instruments, and having relied on them throughout their careers, surgeons often passed them on to the next generation of their families, or bequeathed them to museums.

That tradition ended in the 1930s and 1940s, when ownership of equipment began to shift to clinics and hospitals. Historians worry that as hospitals regard instruments as disposable junk, there will be little left for collections and future documentation.

And there will be much to talk about. While the techniques of grasping, cutting, clamping, removing and joining tissues have remained fairly constant through the ages, 20th century breakthroughs have advanced the field in previously unimaginable ways. Thomas Edison's electric light bulb changed everything, as did surgical microscopes, fiber-optic instruments and the more recent capability to place a tiny camera at the end of a surgical instrument.

But nothing will replace the surgeon's judgment and skill, Rutkow says, adding, "Many new developments are offshoots of computer technology. But, although automation may ultimately robotize the surgeon's hand, the practice of surgery will retain its roots as both a manual art and a science."

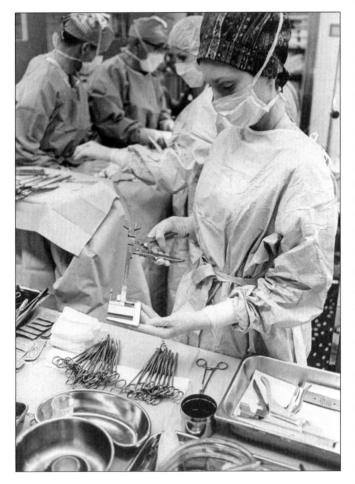

A nurse in this undated photo prepares a surgical stapler, introduced in the United States in 1966.

Source: Corbis-Bettmann/UPI

In War and Peace

Today's Sophisticated Military Hospitals Grew from Makeshift Revolutionary War Units

by Gloria Shur Bilchik

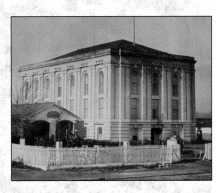

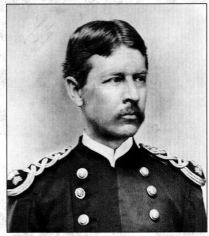

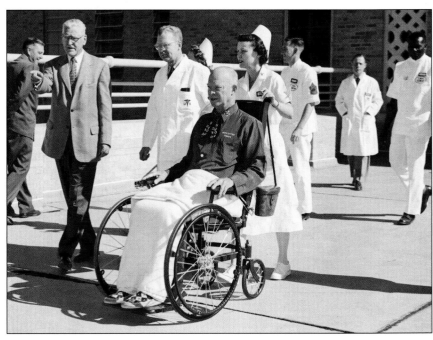

During the Civil War, Union soldiers were treated at the military hospital in Armory Square, Washington, DC (top left, circa 1865). Major Walter Reed (bottom left), an Army surgeon and a U.S. public health commissioner, is credited with finding a cure for yellow fever. In 1907, five years after his death, Congress allocated money for the flagship Army hospital in Washington, DC, that bears Reed's name. President Dwight D. Eisenhower (top) meets the press in October 1955 at Fitzsimmons Army Hospital in Colorado for the first time since suffering a heart attack.

Sources: (clockwise) Corbis/U.S. Army Military History Institute, Corbis/UPI, Corbis-Bettmann

During the decade following World War II, Fitzsimmons Army Hospital was usually a quiet place. Then, on Sept. 25, 1955, President Dwight D. Eisenhower suffered a heart attack while on a fishing vacation in nearby Denver, and Fitzsimmons' serenity was shattered. As Eisenhower was admitted, reporters flocked to the hospital and pressed for information. Phones jangled, consultants and political aides scurried about, and world attention focused on Fitzsimmons as the president convalesced.

Eisenhower's choice of hospitals was hardly random. As a retired five-star Army general, he sought medical care at a hospital representing his branch of service. And because of the way military hospitals had evolved, he could expect to receive treatment equal to that offered by the nation's most famous academic medical centers.

But that evolution spanned many generations. Modern military hospitals and the "M.A.S.H." units fictionalized (and highly exaggerated) by Hollywood have their roots in the Roman Empire, when primitive facilities traveled with soldiers on military campaigns, says Dale C. Smith, chairman of the department of medical history at Uniformed Services University, Bethesda, MD.

Roots in the Revolutionary War

The first American combat hospitals were set up in tents during the Revolutionary War. Makeshift affairs capable of only limited remedial care, their staffs generally consisted of a regimental surgeon (all military doctors were called "surgeons") and a few surgeon's mates, who bathed and fed the patients. "The assistants were soldiers considered expendable by commanding officers," says Smith. "They were the drunks and the stupid. The doctor was expected to cope."

During the same era, an attempt was made to establish permanent military hospitals in New York and Philadelphia, the big cities of the colonies. But staff was hard to come by, and the embattled colonists were having trouble holding on to the cities. So the effort failed. After 1776, the successful American revolutionaries packed up their hospital tents, and military hospitals vanished until they were again needed for the War of 1812.

Meanwhile, in 1798, President John Adams signed the Marine Hospital Act, under which a portion of sailors' monthly pay was set aside for building and staffing hospitals for Marines and seamen. (Later, these facilities evolved into the hospitals of the Public Health Service, which is celebrating its 200th anniversary this year.)

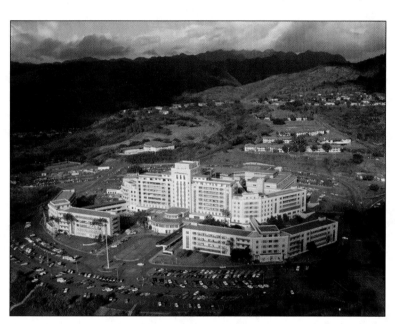

Honolulu's vast Tripler Army Medical Center (1992) shows how military hospitals have grown in size and sophistication.

Source: Corbis/Douglas Peebles

A Port in the Storm
The U.S. Navy began operating hospitals in the 1820s. Hospitals in Norfolk, New Orleans, New York, Philadelphia and Boston were built to accommodate sick and wounded active-duty sailors between cruises. They were among the first permanent military hospitals in the nation.

In the 1890s, the Navy was the first branch of service to institute a training hierarchy for young physicians. In the Army, chief surgeon William Borden pushed hard for a training hospital at Washington Barracks, in the nation's capital. Year after year, he was turned down. Then, in 1907, looking for a way to memorialize Major Walter Reed, M.D., who was considered a hero for finding the cure for yellow fever, Congress allocated money for the flagship Army hospital in Washington, DC, that still bears Reed's name.

State-of-the-art care became the military norm in World War I. In 1915, George Crile, M.D., a civilian physician serving in the Army Reserve, set up a base hospital on the grounds of Case Western Reserve University's medical school in Cleveland. Crile's idea of putting medical school faculty members on reserve to care for soldiers caught on, and soon similar hospitals were established at Harvard, Johns Hopkins and Columbia medical schools. The system worked well, and in World War II, one fully equipped facility operated as the Hospital Ship Solis and was staffed by the University of Pennsylvania's medical school faculty.

After the war, the military's general hospitals established training residencies, again employing medical school faculty reservists as the supervising physicians. "That's when military hospitals really became the equivalent of academic medical centers," Smith says.

A Question of Readiness
Today, according to the Department of Defense,108 military hospitals are in operation, on Army posts, and on naval and air bases in the U.S and abroad. But that number represents a significant decrease, as post-Cold War military downsizing has forced the closing of 23 military hospitals, including Fitzsimmons. However, many familiar names in historically important locations remain—Tripler (Hawaii), Bethesda, Walter Reed, Guantanamo Bay (Cuba). Also still operating is an Army hospital at Fort Gordon, AR, named for Dwight Eisenhower.

Topping the current list of issues facing military hospitals are concerns about funding, quality, managed care and the ability to serve their constituencies. There's also a continuing debate about military medicine's state of readiness for a crisis. One thing, however, is certain: At the end of the 20th century, military hospitals and their civilian counterparts have more in common than ever.

ONE FOOT IN EACH WORLD

Volunteers Forge Vital Links between Hospitals and Communities

by Margaret Castrey

When thousands of wounded GIs came home from World War II, community involvement in hospitals exploded. Volunteers fed patients in traction, pushed wheelchairs across sprawling hospital campuses, and staged entertainments. They performed a myriad of tasks that relieved paid staff and helped patients and their families.

Volunteer numbers surge during any war, but the end of World War II saw the biggest jump in history. With GIs back on the payroll, Rosie the Riveter lost her wartime job and she and her peers headed to local hospitals to volunteer.

Managing these swelling numbers began to require full-time attention, and by 1946, the Veteran's Administration established "director of volunteer services" as a civil-service job category.

The road to that official job description stretches back almost two centuries. In 1752, Ben Franklin volunteered, raising money to build Pennsylvania Hospital for indigent and mentally ill patients. He launched the first matching fund drive and published the first hospital development report, complete with a contribution form on the last page.

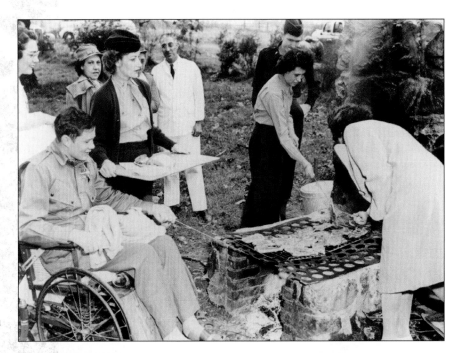

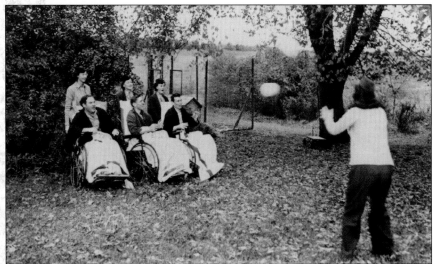

A group of Red Cross volunteers called the Grey Ladies were an essential part of O'Reilly General Hospital, Springfield, MO, during World War II. In these photos, the volunteers hold a barbecue for soldiers being treated at the hospital. O'Reilly was one of the 10 largest Army hospitals in the United States between 1941 and 1946, with 3,500 beds in 253 buildings, and the Grey Ladies were integral to its smooth operation. Throughout the history of American hospitals, volunteers have helped in a variety of tasks, from raising funds to raising patients' spirits.

Courtesy of The History Museum for Springfield-Greene County.

"Women volunteered before Pennsylvania Hospital's doors even opened," says Nancy Brown, executive director of the AHA's Volunteer Administration and Auxiliary Services. "A group of widows and other single women of Philadelphia donated money to have drugs shipped from London for charity patients." Through the centuries, such groups of women continued to raise money, make sheets and infant clothing, greet visitors, and roll bandages.

Doctors' Spouses Help Out

By 1872, doctors had begun to cut back on house calls and instead saw working-class patients in hospitals. "Doctors didn't have time to stay at the bedside, so they asked their wives to drop by the hospital to reassure lonely patients," says Pat Rowell, director of volunteer services at Massachusetts General Hospital, Boston. The physicians' spouses obliged, forming a Ladies Visiting Committee that still exists.

That same year in New York, Louisa Lee Schuyler founded the City Hospital Visiting Committee, which sought to better public hospital conditions. These volunteers were not universally welcome. "One early visitor to Metropolitan Hospital was warned that she would be shot if she stepped onto Welfare Island," reports Sally Rogers of the United Hospital Fund, which now operates the committee. Undeterred, the young volunteer "rowed across the river with a guard holding a shotgun across his knee."

Throughout history, the guns of war have challenged hospital resources. A Pennsylvania Hospital report after World War II described an overworked and undermanned staff. Without a huge corps of volunteers, the report said, some wards would have closed until after the war.

To Coin a Phrase

The first teenage volunteers signed up at Evanston (IL) Hospital soon after the bombing of Pearl Harbor. These girls wore red and white striped pinafores, which led an elderly patient to ask, "Where is my pretty little Candy Striper?"

In the early 1960s, a Manassas, VA, women's club founded a group to help open a new hospital. "Membership in the auxiliary was a prestigious thing, and many doctors' wives belonged," says Carolyn Mosseller, longtime volunteer with Prince William Health System.

Young women worked four-hour shifts, doing everything from answering call bells to making beds and helping with baths. Members also operated a coffee shop, preparing some of the food at home. "They even cooked breakfast for doctors," Mosseller says. "They did everything in order to make things go."

Today, most volunteers are either teenagers or retirees, notes Wendy Biro-Pollard, volunteer director at St. David's Medical Center, Austin, TX. She is researching ways to attract working people. One young adult program interests her because it offers short-term projects, training, flexible schedules, and social activities.

"I'm also searching for a model for an auxiliary-supported day care center," Biro-Pollard says, "so stay-at-home moms can volunteer without paying for a sitter."

Now, volunteers do more than push the flower cart. At St. David's, they help wheelchair-bound patients learn to scuba dive. At VA Western New York Health Care System in Buffalo, they run computers and prepackage medications. At Massachusetts General, volunteers translate medical jargon across many languages.

In this day of high-tech medicine, says Rosemary Fox, chair of the AHA Committee on Volunteers, "Sometimes a volunteer is the only nonthreatening person the patient sees all day."

Although Massachusetts General estimates that services provided by volunteers would cost the hospital $1.3 million a year, Rowell says that another benefit is more important. "When we have these people involved in the life of the institution who have one foot in each world, they ask the questions that hold hospitals accountable," she says.

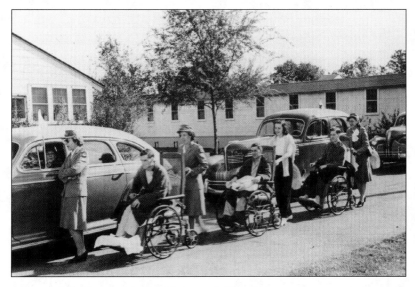

Courtesy of The History Museum for Springfield-Greene County.

THE ENEMY INSIDE

*When Hospital Staffs Started Washing Their Hands,
the Infection War Was On*

by Gloria Shur Bilchik

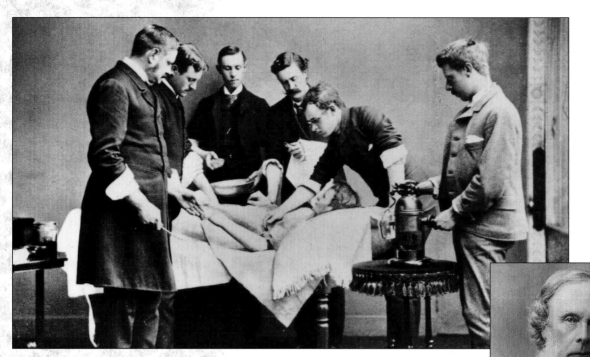

Until antiseptic techniques became the norm, cleanliness was not valued. "Indeed, cleanliness was out of place," wrote Sir Frederick Trewes, in an essay published in the early 1870s. "It was considered to be finicking and affected. The surgeon operated in a slaughter-house-suggesting frock coat of black cloth. The more sodden it was, the more forcibly did it bear evidence to the surgeon's prowess." Surgeons in 1870 Scotland (top photo) used a carbolic acid sprayer to control infections during surgery. The technique was invented by Joseph Lister (right), an early proponent of Louis Pasteur's germ theories and the man some call the father of antisepsis. Source: Corbis/Library of Congress

In 1840s' Vienna, a young physician named Ignac Semmelweis made a world-changing observation. Aware that childbed ("puerperal") fever was killing as many as 25 percent of women in the days following childbirth, Semmelweis found it curious that the deaths occurred almost exclusively among women who delivered their infants in hospitals. Those who delivered at home, and those who self-delivered in alleys and streets, rarely contracted the fatal condition.

Further investigation led Semmelweis to see a link between the standard medical-school curriculum and maternal deaths. Each day, medical students and professors dissected several cadavers, often between patient rounds. Although the concept of germs was as yet undiscovered, "Semmelweis concluded that the transmission of what he called 'invisible cadaver particles' was the cause of childbed fever," says Sherwin B. Nuland, M.D., author of *Doctors, The Biography of Medicine.* "The transmitting source of the 'cadaver particles' was to be found in the hands of the students and attending physicians."

Fearing the Terrible Truth
Semmelweis then instituted the simple measure of washing hands in a chlorine solution. His hygienic practices dramatically reduced the number of deaths caused by childbed fever. But his theory met strong resistance from

established physicians, who were offended by the abrasive upstart and slow to acknowledge the terrible truth that their own entrenched procedures may have caused so many deaths, says Nuland. Semmelweis did not publish his results for another 15 years.

In the 1860s, British physician Joseph Lister broadened the battle to include post-surgical infections, which were almost universal and frequently fatal. Lister was an early adopter of Louis Pasteur's recently postulated germ theory. Learning that a nearby city had eliminated a stench in its sewers by pouring carbolic acid down the drains, he reasoned that the chemical had killed microorganisms like those identified by Pasteur. Applying this conclusion to surgery, he then devised a wound dressing soaked in carbolic acid. Later, he added a sprayer to drench the entire surgical area in a mist of carbolic acid solution.

Soon, Lister began applying it to his hands and instruments. Lister's first report on this treatment was published in *The Lancet* in 1867, the year now regarded as the birth date of antisepsis.

"Listerism" Changes Everything

As "Listerism" gradually gained acceptance, its principles of cleanliness caught on. The surgeon's traditional black frock coat, elegantly tailored, stained with blood and rarely laundered, began to be covered by a rubber apron designed to protect the coat from disinfectant.

Then, in the 1870s and 1880s, surgeons began to move beyond Lister's antiseptic approach. Through newer aseptic procedures, surgeons attempted to exclude infectious bacteria by boiling or heating instruments, sutures, towels and sponges. Increasingly convinced that their own clothing might be a source of infection, some surgeons began to wear loose-fitting gowns over their street clothes. Some, but not all, anesthetists, assistants, and spectators also replaced their street coats with special sterilized cotton or linen coats.

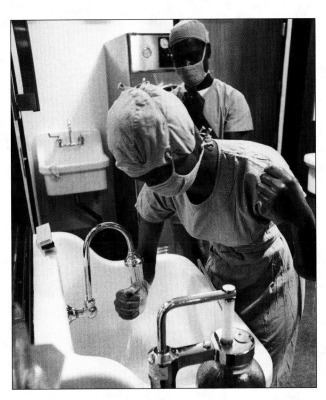

In the mid- and late 1800s, aseptic techniques gradually gained acceptance, and surgical staffs undertook elaborate sterilizing procedures for themselves and their surgical gowns and equipment. In the 1982 photo above, a nurse washes up before surgery at St. Christopher's Hospital, Philadelphia. Source: Corbis/Ed Eckstein

An elaborate ritual of hand washing became the norm, and in 1893, William Halsted became the first surgeon to wear sterile rubber gloves while performing an operation.

By 1910, surgical caps and gloves had become widely accepted. Few surgeons, however, welcomed the advent of face masks. "Early masks, which became quickly saturated with moisture from breathing and talking, irritated surgeons, especially those with beards," says James M. Edmunson, author of *Surgical Garb*. "For these reasons, many surgeons preferred to enforce a rule of silence during operations, rather than don a cumbersome and largely ineffective mask."

Aseptic techniques even influenced operating room decor. By the 1920s, white gowns, starched white linens, and the sparkling white operating room symbolized the modern concept of healing.

No one, however, has yet found a way to completely eliminate hospital-based ("nosocomial") infections. In the 1950s and 1960s, a nationwide pandemic of staphylococcal infection spurred a movement toward systematic infection-control in hospitals. As a result, infection control has emerged as a specialty, and several national organizations dedicate themselves to standard-setting, education and enforcement.

Today, statistics published by the Hospital Infections Program (HIP) of the Centers for Disease Control and Prevention reveal that nosocomial infections affect about 2 million patients each year. HIP studies also indicate that a third of these infections can be prevented by well-organized infection-control programs.

More than a century after the concepts of infection control began to unfold, many challenges remain, says Elaine Larson in a 1997 article published in the *American Journal of Infection Control*. "They await the Semmelweis, the Lister and the Nightingale of our times."

A LIFELINE FOR THE MEDICALLY INDIGENT

30 Years Ago, No One Foresaw How Vital–and Enormous–
Medicaid Would Become

by Margaret Castrey

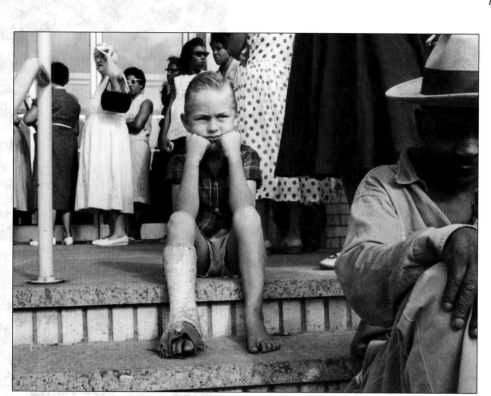

Concerns about children have often driven federal health care programs. In the early 1900s, the Children's Bureau surveyed the status of American youths; its findings helped shape the Shepard-Towner Act of 1920, which established the first federal matching grants to help states pay for physical exams and midwife training. A young man waits none too patiently for doctors to check his broken leg at a Dallas County Hospital clinic in the mid-1900s.

Source: Parkland Health & Hospital System

When President Johnson signed Medicaid into existence in 1965, hardly anybody noticed. Public attention was fixed on the big new Medicare health insurance program. Tiny Medicaid, in contrast, merely tweaked the federal relationship with state programs for the poor. Few people thought it would amount to much.

After all, this was the '60s. "The economy was booming and unemployment was low," recalls Leo Greenawalt, president of the Washington State Hospital Association. "It seemed obvious that most people would get their health coverage at work, and that only the poorest of the poor would ever need Medicaid."

That assumption, of course, proved false. By 1966, some 36 million people turned to Medicaid for assistance.

Medicaid's ancestry harks back to the beginning of this century. Care of the poor had been a local affair until 1912, when a new federal agency, the Children's Bureau, began to investigate the status of children. "The bureau's surveys helped shape the 1920 Shepard-Towner Act," says Rima Apple, professor of human ecology and women's studies at the University of Wisconsin. "That bill set up the first federal matching grants to help states pay for physical examinations and the training of midwives.

"Reformers were pushing for this type of legislation," Apple says. "Most people say it passed because Congress was afraid women who had just gained suffrage would vote as a bloc."

Decades of Expansion

By the 1930s, the Social Security Act extended aid to dependent children. In the 1940s, private insurance expanded rapidly as businesses used health benefits to circumvent wartime wage caps. Public pressure mounted to give better health care to the poor, and in the 1950s and 1960s the federal government gradually expanded its role.

Although the public barely noticed, Medicaid did create a significant change. "With the passage of Medicaid, a whole group of people ceased to be medically indigent," recalls Ruth Rothstein, chief of Chicago's Cook County Bureau of Health Services and director of Cook County Hospital. "They had green insurance cards. We might not like what we received for their care, but they were paid for."

Throughout its history, politicians have wrangled over Medicaid. In 1970, when Howard Newman became Medicaid commissioner, the early prevention, screening, diagnosis and treatment program was not yet reaching its target. Convinced of the importance of the federal role, Newman issued a memo suggesting that state agencies use Head Start to identify and enroll eligible children. After the memo went out, President Nixon began his second term and replaced Health, Education and Welfare Secretary Elliott Richardson with Casper Weinberger, who rescinded the memo. Although a frustrated Newman cited the law and invoked the right thing to do, he was told simply: "It would cost too much."

The 1970s brought increased awareness of needs: nursing home standards, long-term coverage, pregnant women, and children. The expansions continued with two important events for hospitals in 1981: the start of the disproportionate-share program and the passage of the Boren Amendment. "The Boren Amendment was originally intended to give states flexibility," says Molly Collins, senior associate policy director for the AHA. "Then it evolved into a tool hospitals and nursing homes used to challenge the states."

As the 1980s' economy flagged, fewer businesses offered health insurance. Pressure for Medicaid increases

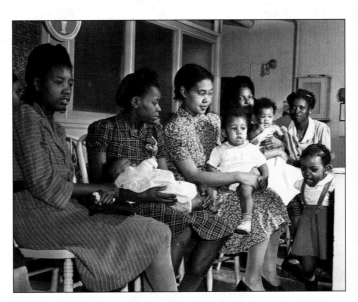

More sanguine mothers watch their children while awaiting their turn to see a doctor at Children's Hospital, Washington, DC, in 1943. President Johnson signed Medicaid into law in 1965; today, children are again the focus. The AHA and others are involved in outreach efforts to sign up children who are eligible for Medicaid. The federal government is encouraging states to expand Medicaid or create other programs to cover kids through the Children's Health Insurance Program.

Source: Corbis/Library of Congress

mounted and enrollment more than doubled between 1988 and 1992. Budgets exploded as states found creative ways to increase their dollar matches.

Meanwhile, the federal role changed dramatically. "Early on, our job was mainly to cajole, encourage, and support the states in doing what they were obliged to do for Medicaid," Newman says. "Over time, the idea of the federal government reviewing and evaluating the states has withered away and the focus has become 'How can we get the most federal money for our program?'"

In reaction to increased costs, Congress sought to reduce Medicaid from entitlement to block grant status in the mid-1990s. Supporters called public attention to the proposal, saying it would unravel the country's only safety net for poor children, the disabled, and Medicare itself.

After 30 years, Medicaid was gaining some visibility. "Before the block grant effort," says one congressional aide, "probably half the people in Congress didn't know Medicare from Medicaid."

This increased attention has not made fulfilling the mission easier, however. In Texas, reports Ron Anderson, M.D., president and CEO of Dallas' Parkland Hospital, at least 60,000 children who are eligible for Medicaid still have not been enrolled.

Money alone cannot provide all the answers. In Illinois, the Hospital and Health Systems Association says its state's initial 1966 appropriation would fund barely a week of current Medicaid costs.

The AHA is making outreach to uninsured children a priority through the Campaign for Coverage . . . a Community Health Challenge, which the association is sponsoring with state, regional, and metropolitan associations. And the federal government is making matching funds available through the Children's Health Insurance Program for states to expand Medicaid or create other programs to cover uninsured children.

"IN THE NAME OF HUMANITY"

Europeans Brought Epidemics to Native Americans, but Help Has Been a Long Time Coming

by Gloria Shur Bilchik

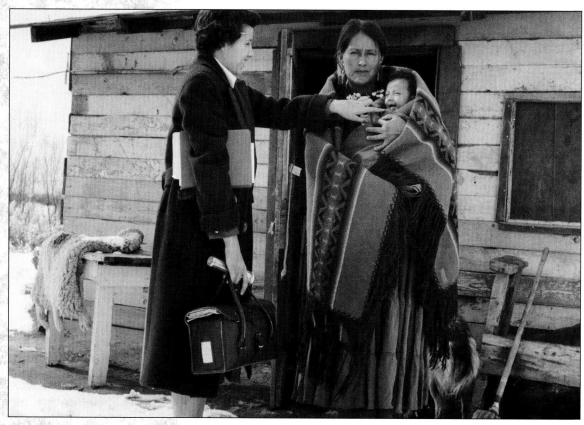

A health care worker visits an Indian woman and her baby on a reservation in 1965.   Source: Corbis-Bettmann

When European explorers first encountered the native tribes of America, they brought along many things the Indians had never seen before—including smallpox, trachoma, measles, influenza, cholera, typhoid and venereal diseases. As a result, Indian populations experienced continuing waves of devastating epidemics, and the health of America's first residents began a downward spiral.

For a while in early U.S. history, the policy of maintaining a separate Indian Country was generally accepted. But by the 1840s, to make way for westward expansion, that notion gave way to the idea of creating reservations.

"Government policy became aimed at 'civilizing' the tribes by destroying native culture and replacing it with the values and practices of white America," says Robert

Trennert, author of *White Man's Medicine: Government Doctors and the Navajo, 1863-1955.*

The effect was further deterioration of Indian health. In the confined, alien environment of the reservation, old methods of nutrition and sanitation disappeared. Traditional means of food production, such as the buffalo hunt, vanished, because Indians were expected to adopt farming. But reservation agriculture seldom produced enough food, leaving the residents vulnerable to starvation and disease.

"A National Disgrace"

Under these circumstances, the government had no choice but to introduce some form of basic health care, says Trennert. Responsibility fell to the U.S. Office of Indian Affairs (OIA). Originally a part of the War

Department, it moved in 1849 to the newly created Department of the Interior.

Meanwhile, Indians continued to acquire white-men's illnesses. Well-meaning military units and missionaries often added to the natives' health problems. "They gave out bacon, coffee and unfamiliar types of beans," Trennert says. "The Indians didn't know how to prepare these foods, so many died from stomach disorders."

By the late 1800s, while health care for other Americans was benefiting from many advancements, reservation Indians still had no hospitals or facilities for treating acute illnesses, accidents or contagious diseases. "These services ought to be furnished them in the name of humanity," then-Indian Commissioner Thomas J. Morgan wrote. "I have been powerless to remedy a great evil, which in my view amounts to a national disgrace."

In 1873, the humanitarian advocacy of Morgan and a number of missionaries paid off. The Office of Indian Affairs established a division to supervise health efforts on reservations and began a field-nurse program. The first federal Indian hospital was built in the 1880s in Oklahoma.

A Slow and Painful Period of Catching Up

But both Indian health services and health status took many years to catch up to contemporary standards. In the 1920s, an Indian facility in New Mexico lacked the money to buy a sterilizer, so its staff made do with a pressure cooker owned by the doctor's wife, writes Eleanor Gregg, author of *Indians and the Nurse.* And as recently as 1953, the incidence of tuberculosis among Indians was five times that found in the general population.

One hero in this otherwise dismal saga was John Collier, who served as commissioner of Indian Affairs in the 1930s. Collier's reformist program created unprece-

dented research and prevention programs, and construction of more hospitals, with the total reaching 93 by 1938.

A major turning point came in 1955, when the U.S. Public Health Service took over responsibility for Indian health. "In the 1950s, there was pressure to eliminate the Bureau of Indian Affairs completely. This move saved Indian health care," Trennert says.

Today, the Indian Health Service (IHS) is the primary source of medical care for approximately 1.34 million American Indian and Alaska Native people. It operates more than 500 health care facilities, including 51 hospitals, and it maintains a separate urban Indian health program, with 12 clinics and 22 community services programs.

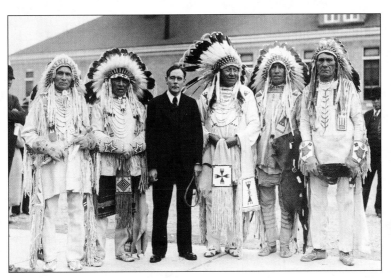

John Collier, the commissioner of Indian Affairs, meets with chiefs of the Blackfoot Indians in Rapid City, SD, in 1934. Collier sought to reverse the federal government's dismal record of health care for native Americans, championing research and prevention programs and overseeing the construction of modern hospitals on reservations. Still, it wasn't until the late 1950s that health care leaders began to consider the traditions and taboos of Indian culture when developing health programs, a sensitivity that continues to evolve. Source: Corbis-Bettmann

Finally, Progress, but a Way to Go

Under the IHS, health status among the nation's more than 545 Indian tribes, bands and villages has increased significantly. Since 1973, infant mortality has decreased by 54 percent, maternal mortality by 65 percent and tuberculosis mortality by 74 percent. Still, health status is not on par with the general U.S. population.

But the IHS is clearly intent on improving the situation. This year, the $168 million Alaska Native Medical Center in Anchorage became the newest IHS facility. Opened in June, the center offers contemporary care in a setting amenable to native traditions: It includes an igloo-like meditation room, and its windows can be unlocked for special ceremonies —to let the spirit escape after a death, for example.

That level of sensitivity has taken a long time to evolve. But the new medical center is emerging as a symbol—a redeeming epilogue in the history of health care for America's first residents. "Natives are owed first-class health care," Alaska's Sen. Ted Stevens said at the center's dedication ceremony. "No one in the future will say that the federal government didn't keep its promise."

Society's Most Vulnerable

Sick Children Often Faced Neglect or Worse,
Until Reformers Stepped In

by Margaret Castrey

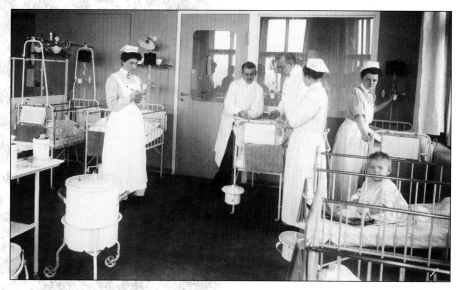 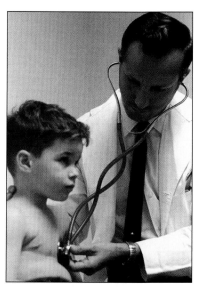

Nurses tend to patients in a ward of New York Children's Hospital (left) circa 1910. Prior to the 19th century, chronically ill or disabled children were often abandoned or even killed by their families, who did not have the wherewithal to care for them. Children's Hospital of Philadelphia opened in 1855 with 12 beds, becoming the first facility of its kind in the United States. In the 1967 photo (right), a doctor examines a boy at Kaiser Hospital, Oakland.

Sources: Corbis-Bettmann (left), Corbis/Ted Streshinsky (right)

When a saloonkeeper noticed a woman trying to give away her crippled 5-year-old daughter near the Kansas City stockyards in the summer of 1887, he sent word to dentist Alice Graham. Together with her sister, Katharine Richardson, M.D., Graham searched the area and found the child, abandoned. They took the girl to a small maternity hospital and established the Free Bed Fund Association that evolved into Children's Mercy Hospital.

The fact that people would care about an abandoned girl showed that society's attitudes toward children were changing. When 19th century reformers appeared on the scene, "sick children were frequently abandoned and infanticide was a common practice," writes Geneva Katz, historian for the National Association of Children's Hospitals and Related Institutions.

Families that did care kept sick children "at home because most infants and many children admitted to adult hospitals died of cross infection, diarrhea, or neglect," writes Shirley Bonnem in her history of The Children's Hospital of Philadelphia. Poor staffing and lack of infection controls made a hospital a very dangerous place.

Children of this era succumbed readily to epidemic yellow fever, scarlet fever, measles, diphtheria, smallpox, typhoid, typhus, cholera and whooping cough, and were crippled by bone and joint infections. But reformers and philanthropists sought to change that.

Another First for Philadelphia

The first European children's facility opened in Paris in 1802. Half a century later, a newly trained American physician, Francis Lewis, M.D., visited London's new Hospital for Sick Children. He was so taken with the concept, he brought the model home. In 1855, he and two other physicians opened America's first facility, the Children's Hospital of Philadelphia.

Although men established that first one, most subsequent children's hospitals were founded, supported and directed by women.

With just 12 beds, Lewis' hospital depended on its large dispensary to provide outreach. In truth, early inpatient care could offer little more than a brace or better food and the hope that children would get better, says Dr. Charles Rosenberg, author of *The Care of Strangers: The Rise of America's Hospital System.*

Gradually, technical practice began to play a larger role. Medicine evolved techniques for antiseptic surgery, began to understand infectious disease, and developed sophisticated orthopedic procedures, clinical labs and X-rays. Yet, medical professionals and dedicated philanthropists could have accomplished little without the support of their communities.

Community Help Is Vital

At Children's Mercy, a sign out front contained a sliding blackboard. "If Dr. Richardson put on the sign that she needed sheets, people going to work would get them to her," says archivist Carol Belt, R.N. Families with big vegetable gardens donated home-canned foods and a nearby dairy sent a wagon with milk, cream and eggs.

Through the years, families and celebrities of every stripe have helped pay the bills. Children's Hospital of Philadelphia, says Bonnem, is said to have benefited when gangster Al Capone sent a $1,000 check from his jail cell.

In the 1930s, children's hospitals helped legitimize pediatrics as a specialty by appointing pediatrics professors to staff positions. As associations like the American Academy of Pediatrics were founded and certification procedures developed, pediatricians gradually took over the care of sick children from general practitioners.

Children's hospitals themselves evolved to meet local needs. Freestanding acute care hospitals like Children's Mercy often developed nursing schools to train staff.

As medical care began to save more children from illness and injury, the need for a second type of hospital grew. St. Mary's Hospital for Children, Bayside, NY, eliminated acute care to specialize instead in evaluation and rehabilitation for convalescence.

A third type of hospital came to reside within a larger academic medical institution or hospital system. For example, the Floating Hospital in Boston, initially a boat that took patients sailing, in 1931 joined with Tufts University to become the New England Medical Center.

Advances That Astound

Today's well-funded, technology-rich hospitals would amaze caregivers from previous eras. Belt was a student nurse in the 1940s. She remembers overworked nurses diapering infants in red and white checked towels when cloth diapers ran low, sharpening needles on a whetstone, and patching, powdering and sterilizing rubber gloves.

"We had 14 cribs to a ward and used a relay system to wash the babies in a cast-iron sink," Belt recalls. "We all took turns in the formula lab, filling small-necked bottles and sterilizing them in the autoclave down the hall. Before IV fluids, we used to mix salt and water and run it through tubing into great long needles under the skin to get babies re-hydrated."

Continuing medical advances expanded the children's hospital repertoire: advanced surgery, intensive care, home care, and treatment of disability, disfigurement, cancer, congenital heart defects and trauma. Today, all are eminently treatable.

When the first American hospital was established, children had neither medical nor social importance. Today, more than 150 members of the National Association of Children's Hospitals and Related Institutions bear witness to a modern idea: children are a most precious resource.

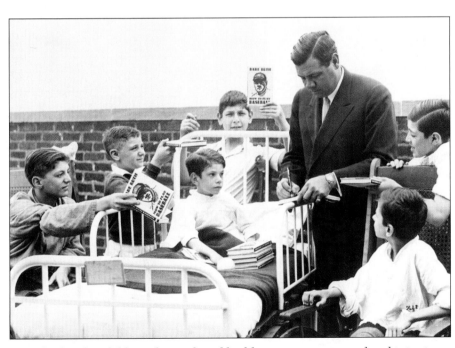

Over the decades, children's hospitals and health care grew in size and sophistication thanks to health care reformers and celebrities who helped raise attention, funds and the spirits of the young patients. Babe Ruth signs autographs for youngsters at a New York City hospital in 1931. Source: Corbis-Bettmann

THE ART OF DYING

In Its Brief History, Hospice Has Become a Welcome Option in the Continuum of Life

by Gloria Shur Bilchik

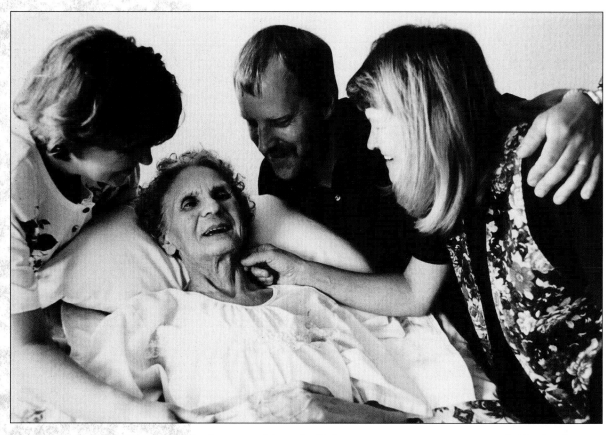

Among hospice goals is to make the family a part of the end-of-life experience. A patient is surrounded by family members and hospice staff.   Photo courtesy of NHO.

Although the first American hospice specializing in care for dying patients opened in 1974, the concept is far from new. In the ancient Tibetan Book of the Dead, readers received guidance about how to die consciously, in a state of spiritual enlightenment. A medieval Christian text describes Ars Moriendi, the art of dying. And historians have documented the existence of special homes and facilities for end-of-life care in ancient Rome and Syria.

The Latin word "hospes" meant both host and guest. For hundreds of years, "hospice" was a familiar word,

referring to a house of rest and entertainment for pilgrims, travelers or strangers, and for the destitute or the sick.

"In medieval times, dying persons were seen as prophetic souls," wrote Sandol Stoddard, in *The Hospice Movement: A Better Way of Caring for the Dying*. "They were voyagers and pilgrims valuable to the community in a number of ways, not least in the opportunity they provided those around them for service and spiritual growth."

So it was logical when, in the early 1960s, Cicely Saunders, M.D., adopted the term "hospice" as the name for a new program she was establishing at St. Christopher's in London. Her approach charted new directions in both philosophy and techniques for treating terminally ill patients.

"The name was chosen because this will be something between a hospital and a home, with the skills of one and the hospitality, warmth and the time of the other," Saunders said.

Soon afterwards, Saunders was invited to visit Yale University to lecture to medical students, nurses, social workers and chaplains on her concept of holistic hospice care.

"You matter because you are you," Saunders is said to have explained to her hospice patients. "You matter to the last moment of your life, and we will do all we can not only to help you die peacefully, but also to live until you die."

First in the United States

Saunders' presentations inspired Florence Wald, then dean of the Yale School of Nursing, to take a sabbatical to work at St. Christopher's to learn everything she could about hospice.

In 1974, Wald helped found the Connecticut Hospice in Branford, the first in the United States. Regarded as the role model for many hospices that followed, the 44-bed facility operated in a former private home, with hospice-trained nurses and physicians, and a homelike atmosphere for families and friends.

But acceptance of the hospice concept was not automatic. "The idea ran against the current. American-style medicine had little interest in tending to the needs of the dying or of their families," says Bill Lamers, M.D., founder of The Hospice of Marin (CA), the first on the West Coast. "Over time, though, hospice has made a seminal contribution to the science of pain and symptom management. That development has helped convert many physicians."

Funding for hospices has evolved gradually, too. The first legislation to provide federal funds for hospices was introduced in 1974 by Sens. Frank Church of Idaho and Frank Moss of Utah. It failed. Then, in 1982, Congress created a Medicare hospice benefit, which became permanent in 1986—the same year that states were first allowed to include hospice in their Medicaid programs.

Now Part of Mainstream Health Care

Today, coverage for hospice also is provided to more than 80 percent of employees in medium and large businesses.

Eighty-two percent of managed care plans offer hospice services, and most private insurance plans include a hospice benefit.

Hospice now is recognized as part of the expected continuum of care. A recent Gallup poll indicated that 90 percent of Americans, if faced with a terminal illness, would prefer to be cared for and die in their homes.

According to the National Hospice Organization, more than 3,000 hospices operate in the United States, serving an estimated 495,000 patients in 1997. More than 90 percent of hospice care hours are provided in patients' homes. And although the hospice movement was at first mostly for cancer patients, it has expanded to include patients with heart disease, lung ailments, AIDS, Alzheimer's disease and virtually any other terminal condition.

The lessons learned have been profound. "Hospice patients have taught me that dying is, most simply, a part of living. When pain is adequately controlled, the time of dying can be a time of remarkable possibilities," wrote Ira Byock, M.D., president of the American Academy of Hospice and Palliative Medicine, in a 1997 article in *The Wall Street Journal*. "The best hospice programs have shown that in addition to being practical and cost-effective, end-of-life care can also help people feel dignified, worthy and loved. We should settle for no less."

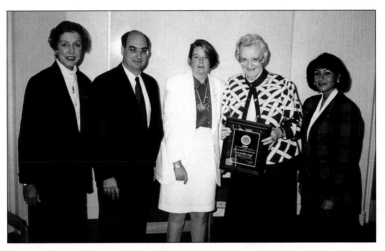

Dame Cicely Saunders (second from right, in photo above), who founded the modern hospice movement in London in the 1960s, receives the Founders Award from the National Hospice Organization (NHO) in 1992. Among NHO officials honoring her were (from right) Samira Beckwith, Margaret Gilmour, John J. Mahoney and Ann MacGregor. Mahoney was NHO president from 1984 to 1998.

Photo courtesy of John J. Mahoney.

INDISPENSABLE

*From Ancient Babylonia to the Computer Age, Pharmacists
Have Served as the Guardians of the Drug Chain*

by Gloria Shur Bilchik

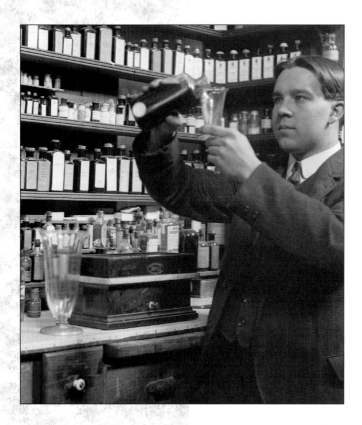

Emil King prepares medicine at his pharmacy in Fulda, MN, in 1905. Although the first American hospital pharmacy was established in 1752 at The Pennsylvania Hospital in Philadelphia, most pharmacists operated out of corner drugstores for the next 200 years. In 1921, only 500 of the 6,000 hospitals in the United States had pharmacists on staff, according to the American Pharmaceutical Association. That began to change in the 1930s and 1940s, and although automation and mail-order services are rapidly changing hospital pharmacy practices, experts believe individual pharmacists will remain critical to monitoring the safe dispensing of drugs.

Source: Corbis/Minnesota Historical Society

Somewhere in prehistory, cave dwellers discovered the soothing benefits of applying cool water, leaves or mud to wounds and sores. Those crude beginnings marked the origin of the science of pharmacy, which historians trace through ancient Babylonia, Egypt, China and Rome.

Some contemporary medicines derive from sources as simple and elementary as those within reach of early man. And many early developments in pharmacy proved enduring, such as Galen's (130–200 A.D.) principles of preparing and compounding medicine, which predominated in the western world for 1,500 years.

Medieval Arab pharmacists made many important contributions to the science, writes George A. Bender, in *Great Moments in Pharmacy*. The first privately owned drugstores were established in Baghdad during the late 8th century. Later, Avicenna, a Persian pharmacist, poet, philosopher and diplomat of the 10th century, developed techniques that were accepted as authority in the West until the 17th century, and still are dominant influences in the Orient.

In colonial America, Christopher Marshall, an Irish immigrant, established one of the first apothecary shops, in Philadelphia in 1729. According to Bender, Marshall's pioneering pharmaceutical enterprise became a leading retail store, a nucleus of large-scale chemical manufacturing, a practical training school for pharmacists, and an important supply depot during the American Revolution. Later, it was managed by Marshall's granddaughter, Elizabeth, America's first woman pharmacist.

America's first hospital pharmacy was established in 1752 at The Pennsylvania Hospital. Jonathan Roberts, an apprentice physician, was hired to arrange medicines and other supplies shipped from London. "Like most other early American hospital apothecaries, Roberts was expected not only to run his shop, but to go on rounds, run the hospital's library, and do minor surgery, such as pulling teeth," says Gregory J. Higby, director of the American Institute of the History of Pharmacy.

Roberts was succeeded by John Morgan, a physician, who was influential in making the established European practice of writing prescriptions a recognized American custom. Morgan also pushed for the official separation of pharmacy from the practice of medicine, arguing that physicians should write prescriptions and that pharmacists should compound and dispense the medications. He believed that this structure would discourage over-drugging. His effort failed for several reasons, Higby says. "Patients chafed under the increased expense and inconvenience. Also, physicians didn't want to give up their pharmaceutical practices, because they relied heavily on the fees they received for the medicines they prescribed."

The profession received a boost in 1821 with the formation of the Philadelphia College of Pharmacy, which was followed closely by similar associations and schools in Massachusetts (1823) and New York (1829). But, according to Glenn Sonnedecker, author of *The History of Pharmacy*, it took the establishment of the American Pharmaceutical Association in 1852 to foster a general professional feeling among pharmacists, and to delineate, once and for all, the border between medicine and pharmacy in the United States.

Until the 1920s, pharmacists remained predominantly entrepreneurs, operating in a corner-drugstore mode. In 1921, the American Pharmaceutical Association estimated that only 500 of the 6,000 hospitals in the United States had pharmacists on staff.

The main reason for hiring a hospital pharmacist in the 1920s was Prohibition. "Medicinal alcohol was still com-

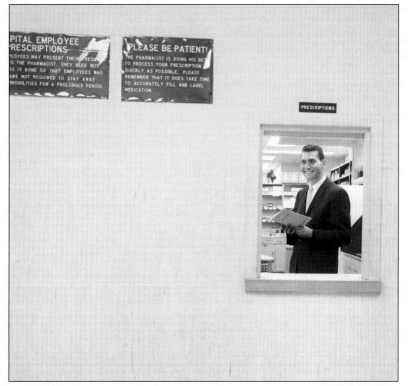

Robert Leventhal is framed by the pharmacy service window at Montefiore Hospital in New York City in 1961. As director, Leventhal pioneered round-the-clock service and quick delivery, turning the Montefiore pharmacy into one of the busiest in New York City.   Source: Corbis-Bettmann

monly prescribed, and a pharmacist provided needed inventory control," Higby says. "Plus, high taxes on alcohol used in commercial preparations made these products expensive. Hospitals could obtain their alcohol tax-free and have their pharmacists manufacture the tinctures, elixirs and fluid extracts that physicians often prescribed in those days."

Once on staff, the pharmacist's role grew—manufacturing much of the hospital's stock preparations, including ointments, syrups, suppositories and tablets. In addition, pharmacists became responsible for making photographic solutions for radiology, pathology and cardiography, and even for ordering surgical instruments and supplies. In the 1930s and 1940s, hospital pharmacists took on the role of "standard-bearers" for the profession, associating themselves with university hospitals and leading the way in raising requirements for hospital practice.

Since then, the importance of hospital pharmacy has continued to grow amid sweeping changes in the pharmaceutical industry. Manufacturing, distribution and dispensing—once the domain of the ancient apothecary and the more modern druggist—now are on the verge of being completely industrialized and robotized. In addition, broader use of technicians and mail-order services are rapidly changing hospital pharmacy practices.

But the individual pharmacist still matters, Higby says. "Health care institutions rely on professional pharmacists as a check on the accuracy of prescriptions, as safeguards in the drug chain, as educators, and as monitors of the proper use of drugs," he says. "The challenge is to ensure that pharmaceutical practitioners, not bottom-line focused corporate managers, guide how medicines are used in the future."

HOSPITALS' CONSCIENCES

*Aunt Ida and Other Pioneers Brought Social Work
Inside the Institution*

by Gloria Shur Bilchik

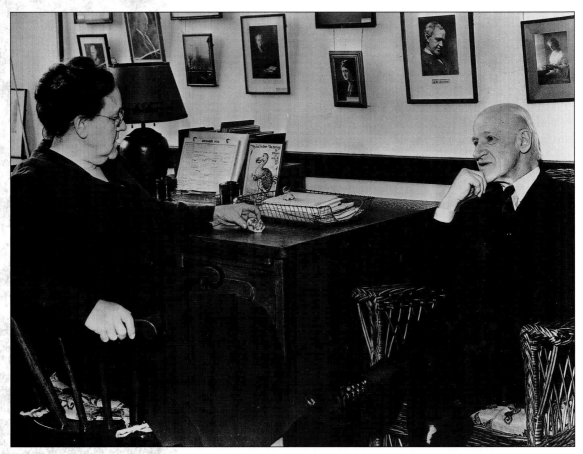

Dr. Richard Cabot confers with Ida Maud Cannon in her office at Massachusetts General Hospital (undated photo). In 1905, Cabot became the first person to invite volunteer social workers into a hospital to help patients. A year later, he enlisted Cannon to set up a department of social work at Massachusetts General. On Cannon's desk is a picture of the dodo bird from "Alice in Wonderland," whose motto she adopted: "The best way to explain it is to do it."   Source: Massachusetts General Hospital

Hospital social work got its start in a place dubbed "The Corner." In 1905, behind a screen in a busy corridor in the outpatient department of Massachusetts General Hospital, a group of social work volunteers set up shop at a few small tables. Their job was to help patients understand their prescriptions and to overcome family and social obstacles to their care as they returned home.

Social workers had never been allowed in hospitals, but these volunteers were invited by Dr. Richard Cabot.

"Cabot was troubled because family and economic problems often interfered with his patients' medical treatment," wrote Harold Lewis, in *Milestones in Social Work and Medicine*. "He welcomed social workers into hospital staffs as possible aides in the management of the social aspects of illness."

Cabot's innovation blended two late-19th century trends: hospital care and the social reform movement. By the late 1800s, "social work" was a well-entrenched term. Services for indigent sick people led the way: In 1853,

Elizabeth Blackwell, a physician, opened a dispensary that evolved into the New York Infirmary for Women and Children. In 1866, she appointed Rebecca Cole, an African-American physician, as a "Sanitary Visitor," who visited the homes of discharged patients. In 1893, Jane Addams organized a dispensary at Hull House Settlement.

After a year of experimentation, Cabot enlisted one of his original volunteers, Ida Maud Cannon, to set up a department of social work in the hospital—the first of its kind in America. Cannon added an unexpected, but lasting twist to the pioneering social work department by helping physicians understand the community from which patients came and the context in which their treatment took place.

The notion of hospital social work quickly took hold in other leading institutions, focusing on the effort to understand and help the individual patient. The 1906 annual report of New York's Mount Sinai Hospital, for example, gave permanent budget support to social services, saying, "The condition of a patient's family while he is in our wards, as well as his needs immediately after discharge, constitute a vital part of his ability to recover and to retain his health."

By 1917, a survey reported 309 paid medical social workers in 17 states, 35 cities and 118 hospitals. Hospital social workers of this era often served as friendly visitors for discharged patients. One case history from the 1900s documents a social worker's role as visiting the patient frequently to encourage her "to not dwell on her problems and to cultivate happy thoughts."

But early on, to the chagrin of those using skill and ingenuity to help patients, the idea that anyone could do medical social work was prevalent. So, social workers

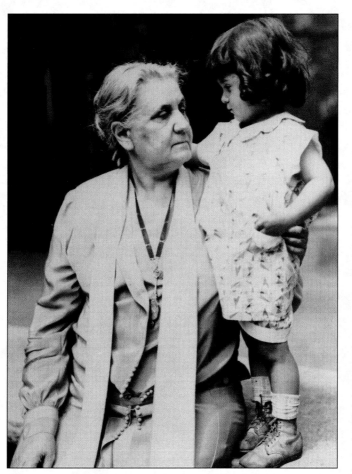

In this 1930 photo, Jane Addams greets a youngster at the 40th anniversary celebration of Hull House in Chicago, which she founded. Source: Corbis-Bettmann

began an effort to create a national, professional organization, and in 1918, the American Association of Hospital Social Workers was established.

"We were a rather motley lot so far as professional preparation was concerned," wrote Cannon, whose warmth, candor and seminal work on behalf of the profession earned her the affectionate nickname "Aunt Ida." "We had come from nursing, teaching, social work and a variety of life experiences. I believe our focus was clear, although our ideas of function and suitable preparation for our work were certainly hazy, to say the least."

Today, the link with the original vision remains strong, and social workers continue their traditional roles in discharge planning, crisis intervention and supportive counseling in acute care. But hospital social work also has expanded in ways that Cannon and her contemporaries could not have imagined, says Rose Popovich, president of the Society of Social Work Leadership in Health Care. "We're case managers, providers of alternative therapies, employee-assistance counselors and behavioral health therapists. We work in emergency rooms, home health care and extended care facilities, as well as settings that weren't even invented until recently—managed care organizations, human resource departments, education and organization development."

Ida Cannon believed that her new profession represented an evolution of hospitals from clinical, professional and economic enterprises to socially aware institutions. "Hospital social service is the tangible evidence of the working of the social conscience in the hospital," wrote Cannon. "Its influence is likely to spread beyond the institution and make contributions to medicine, to nursing and to general social work."

A CENTURY OF THE AHA

Article by Michael Lesparre, former director of the Division of Communications in the AHA's Washington office, with contributions from Gail Lovinger and Kathy Poole, Office of the Secretary, and the AHA Resource Center.

Wrecking crews long ago demolished Cleveland's Colonial Hotel, where eight hospital administrators met in 1899 to found the Association of Hospital Superintendents of the United States and Canada. The group's name has vanished, too—just seven years later, it became the American Hospital Association. But the AHA's mission has stayed the same for 100 years. Today's aim to improve the health of individuals and communities harks back to early missions that spoke about "promoting the welfare of the people."

At the first meeting, the objective was to talk shop about management, economics, hospital inspections, and operating plans. But the founders soon realized they couldn't get far without acknowledging a far more basic interest. "The hospital is an institution in which

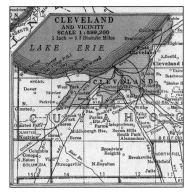

Founded in Cleveland
At the city's Colonial Hotel in September 1899, eight hospital superintendents from Michigan, Ohio, and Pennsylvania met to launch a national association for exchanging ideas. Seven years later, it was renamed the American Hospital Association.

Source: Colliers Encyclopedia

relationships between administrators and nursing supervisors, early meetings focused on care for the poor and indigent. Even hospital food made the agenda. As for professional standards, the association recommended university training in hospital administration for chief executives. To deepen the management ranks, the AHA's 1906 convention voted to admit associate members—those next in line of authority below the superintendent. By 1913, AHA membership included trustees, medical staffs, and superintendents of nursing. Five years later it established institutional membership, and by the time the AHA turned 27, it had 734 members.

As the founders hinted, the link between hospitals and their communities has been strong all along. As early as 1907, records emphasized that the AHA was established to promote better hospital care for all people—

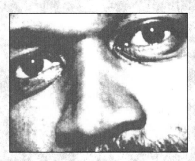

Health Care for All
As early as 1907, racial discrimination made the agenda. Records emphasize that the AHA was founded to promote better hospital care for all people. Members have affirmed this position many times, notably in a 1970 statement on health care for the disadvantaged.

Source: Bettmann Archives

the patient comes first," declared Cincinnati Hospital chief John Fehrenbatch, AHA president in 1903. "His interests and welfare are paramount."

Membership grew to 234 within eight years. Standards and skill building were top concerns, but policy questions were there from the start, too. Along with dispensary abuse, housekeeping, and

and the issue of racial discrimination was on the table. Accountability to the public was considered an official principle of service and fiscal responsibility in 1909. Yet, in some ways, the young organization was very insular. In discussing a paper on hospitals and the political scene, for example, members concluded "that politics and hospitals should not be related at all."

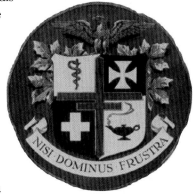

Emblem Trouble
This insignia, now part of the AHA seal, became official in 1927 after an earlier proposal failed to fly. "Very beautiful effects can be produced by embroidering this insignia," gushed the Bulletin of the AHA.

Made possible in part by educational grants from BlueCross BlueShield Association and Fisher HealthCare/A Fisher Scientific Company.

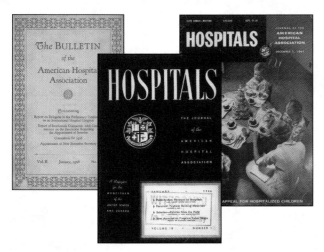

Covering the Field
After running meeting agendas and notices in the National Hospital Record *and elsewhere for many years, the association entered the publishing field in the 1920s, first producing the* Bulletin of the AHA *(shown here in 1928).* Hospitals, *a twice-monthly magazine, made its debut in 1936. With an expanded scope and audience, it was renamed* Hospitals & Health Networks *in 1993.*

Publications weren't as complex at the turn of the century as they are today, but they paralleled the association's development and are a critical part of its history. Magazines and journals carried meeting announcements and agendas, and as hospital management issues began to gel, journal sections were devoted to hospital departments and operations. The AHA used *The National Hospital Record*, which eventually became the independent *Modern Hospital*, as its first official organ. Del Sutton, publisher of the *Record*, was invited to the first meeting as an observer. In the mid-1930s, the AHA began publishing its own magazine, *Hospitals*, which later evolved into

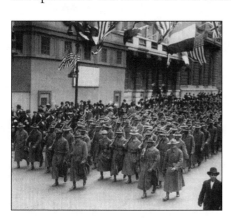

World War I
The association took some of its first steps into public policy during "the war to end all wars." In 1917, it convened a war service committee for hospitals. The AHA urged hospitals and the government to work together in caring for soldiers and attending to the public's welfare.

Source: Bettmann Archives

today's *Hospitals & Health Networks*, and joined the Internet revolution with its home page in 1996.

As the United States entered World War I, the AHA began to get involved in public policy. In 1917, it unanimously passed a resolution to set up a war service committee for hospitals and urged cooperation between hospitals and the government in the care of soldiers and the "health of our people." In the early 1920s, the AHA began working with other national groups to set standards for hospitals and medical education, cooperating with the American College of Surgeons and the American Medical Association. Eventually that cooperation led the groups to set up the Joint Commission on Accreditation of Hospitals, now the Joint Commission on Accreditation of Healthcare Organizations, in 1952.

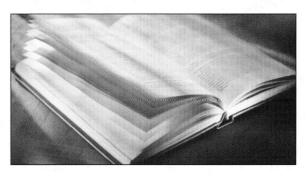

Research Hub
After the war, the Hospital Library and Service Bureau opened and was later acquired by the AHA. Now known as the AHA Resource Center, it houses the Center for Hospital and Healthcare Administration History and the National Information Center for Health Services Administration.

During the postwar years, the Hospital Library and Service Bureau opened at the AHA, though it was initially run by a separate group. The AHA acquired the bureau in 1929. The AHA library and its services to members and other organizations grew rapidly during the next several decades. The library was named for Asa S. Bacon, who had been AHA treasurer for 34 years, president in 1923, and the first chairman of

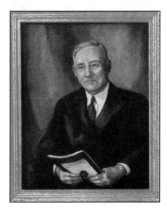

Library Pioneer
The AHA's library was originally named for Asa S. Bacon, its treasurer for 34 years, chairman in 1923, and first head of the standing library committee.

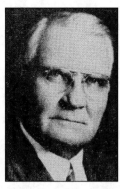

Justin Ford Kimball
He set up the first hospital prepayment plan in Dallas, the prototype for Blue Cross plans. An AHA award for health care financing and delivery honors him.

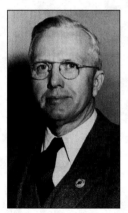

C. Rufus Rorem
An advocate of prepaid coverage, he joined the staff in 1929. The AHA later created the Hospital Service Plan Commission, which became Blue Cross & Blue Shield.

the standing library committee. Now known as the AHA Resource Center, the library houses the Center for Hospital and Healthcare Administration History and the National Information Center for Health Services Administration, created in 1997 by the AHA, the American College of Healthcare Executives, the American College of Physician Executives, and the Healthcare Financial Management Association.

The AHA was an early supporter of health insurance, which made its first appearances in the late 1920s. Justin Ford Kimball had recently organized the first hospital prepayment plan for Dallas teachers in 1929, when the AHA hired C. Rufus Rorem, Ph.D., a nationally recognized proponent of prepaid coverage, as its expert on group hospital insurance. With the support of his colleague, John R. Mannix, assistant director of the University Hospitals of Cleveland, Rorem was largely responsible for Blue Cross insurance as a national movement.

By 1937, the AHA had organized the Hospital Service Plan Commission, which adopted a generic blue cross for its logo and later became Blue Cross and Blue Shield. The AHA also opened associate membership to not-for-profit prepayment plans. Within a year, 40 Blue Cross plans had signed up.

As the AHA became more sensitive to the relationship between the federal government and hospitals, it joined with the Catholic and Protestant hospital associations in

A Letter from FDR
Before there was Hospital Week, there was Hospital Day, as acknowledged in this 1935 letter from Franklin Delano Roosevelt.

1937 to form a joint advisory committee to consider federal legislation and represent the concerns of the field to Congress. Since then, the AHA's advocacy efforts have always emphasized collaboration.

As the association took a greater role on the national scene in the 1930s, big changes occurred internally. It moved out of the space it had shared with *Modern Hospital* and bought a permanent headquarters building at 18 East Division in Chicago. Members founded the House of Delegates to promote a democratic process and formed councils to set standards and create common ground for an increasingly diverse membership. The first councils looked at administrative practice, professional practice, hospital planning and plant operation, public education, government regulations, and association development. AHA members and staff began setting guidelines for working with local governments and insurers. They developed manuals for hospital pharmacies, contracts with doctors, and job descriptions.

Institutional membership became the primary way to belong to the AHA, though personal membership continued. In 1938, the mission underwent a revision: "Its object shall be to promote the welfare of the people through the development of hospital and outpatient services." At the AHA's urging, state and local hospital associations also began to emerge. The Ohio Hospital Association had already opened its doors in 1920 and agreed to collect dues on behalf of the AHA from its constituent members. Soon after, groups formed in Wisconsin, Michigan, and other states.

The association's sharper focus on institutional issues also raised the stakes for chief executives. In 1932, AHA president Paul H.

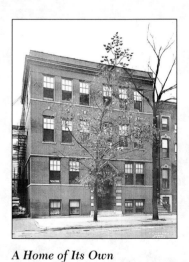

A Home of Its Own
In 1937, the association bought permanent headquarters at 18 East Division Street in Chicago. The same year, members founded the House of Delegates and various standing councils to set policy and standards.

Source: Robert McCullough

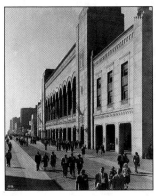

On the Boardwalk
The AHA's 1937 convention in Atlantic City drew 4,091 people from the U.S., Canada, Japan, China, Korea, Cuba, Peru, and elsewhere. Eleanor Roosevelt browsed the exhibit hall, and governors from 21 states, who were holding their own meeting nearby, also stopped by.

Source: Fred Hess & Sons

Fesler, superintendent of Wesley (now Northwestern) Memorial Hospital in Chicago, called for a college of hospital administration modeled after the American College of Surgeons. Within a year, Fesler and others drew up plans for the independent American College of Hospital Administrators and in 1934 presented them to the AHA Board of Trustees. Though the relationship between the two groups would be close, the "AHA could not, by virtue of its own constituency, show any distinction of standards of competency for hospital administrators," the documents stated.

Also in the 1930s, the AHA created awards for leadership and achievements in hospital administration and community service, presenting its first Award of Merit to Matthew O. Foley, editor of *Hospital Management* magazine, in 1934. The 1939 recipient was Malcolm T. MacEachern, M.D., who organized the hospital standards program of the American College of Surgeons. In 1955, the Award of Merit was renamed the Distinguished Service Award.

lished its first *Listing of Hospitals* in 1945, which continues today as the *AHA Guide to the Health Care Field.*

During World War II, the AHA also opened the Wartime Services Bureau to see that members had adequate supplies during shortages and

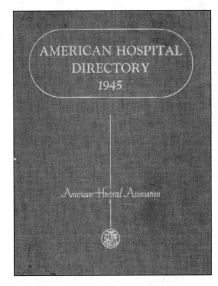

Who They Are, Where They Are
In 1945, the association issued the first Listing of Hospitals, *the forerunner of today's* AHA Guide to the Health Care Field.

Where Credit Is Due
Magazine editor Mathew O. Foley (right) was the first recipient of the Award of Merit in 1934. It was renamed the Distinguished Service Award in 1955.

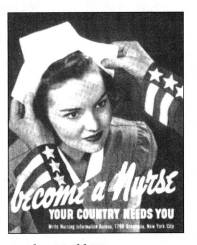

Another World War
With doctors, nurses, and other health professionals joining the armed forces by the thousands, the AHA supported the Cadet Nurse Corps and other efforts to draw women into nursing careers.

The New Deal forever changed perceptions about the federal government's influence on hospitals. With members already reeling from bad debt and renovation needs that languished during the Great Depression, the AHA expanded its advocacy role, joining with the Catholic and Protestant hospital associations to oppose a crush of federal rules and to stress the need for local control over health care. In 1943, recognizing the demands of the AHA's work in the national arena, the board quadrupled membership dues for hospitals—over the protests of AHA CEO Bert Caldwell, who worried that members could not afford the hike. The AHA pub-

rationing. The AHA urged the government to use civilian hospitals for its needs. It also supported the Cadet Nurse Corps in 1943, as thousands of doctors, nurses, dietitians, and other professionals joined the armed forces. The AHA Washington Bureau helped implement the Lanham Act of 1941, which brought federal aid to defense areas, including assistance to nonfederal hospitals. And it teamed up with the U.S. Public Health Service and national nursing groups in urging young women to enter nursing careers.

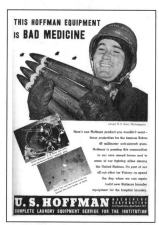

Everybody's War
Even laundry equipment makers were among health care suppliers pressed into wartime service, as seen in this 1944 ad from Hospitals. *The AHA's Wartime Services Bureau helped distribute federal aid to hospitals in defense areas and made sure that shortages and rationing didn't deprive hospitals of critical supplies.*

When the war ended, the association needed little convincing about opening a permanent office in the nation's capital. The wartime bureau was renamed the Washington Service Bureau and was soon steeped in national health policy. Under the leadership of George Bugbee, who succeeded Caldwell as CEO, the AHA helped draft the Hill-Burton Hospital Survey and Construction Act of 1946. Its implementation continued until 1975, and the law remains one of the most significant national events in health care. In the years leading up to Hill-Burton, the AHA's Commission on Hospital Care carried out a national survey that was, in great part, the impetus for the law. Over its 30-year span, Hill-Burton distributed $4 billion to 6,900 hospitals, skilled nursing facilities, nursing homes, and other facilities.

The AHA also supported the National Health Service bill to help the medically indigent, promote health insurance, and extend Social Security benefits to employees of not-for-profit groups. But the association joined other health care groups in opposing mandatory national health insurance, a campaign led by Sen. Robert Wagner of New York. Under pressure from health care associations and others, the Wagner-Murray-Dingell bill fell to defeat. In 1947, the AHA became embroiled in disagreements over a plan by the Veterans Administration to open facilities with more than 150,000 hospital beds. The AHA wanted the government to work with private hospitals to care for veterans, but politics dictated otherwise.

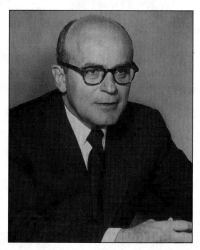

George Bugbee
On his watch as chief executive, the AHA opened a permanent Washington office, pushed for passage of the Hill-Burton Act, and stepped up member services.

Rising costs and access to care increasingly appeared on the radar screen in the 1940s, leading to calls for voluntary health insurance. During Bugbee's tenure as CEO, the AHA created the Blue Cross Commission and the Council on Prepayment Plans and Hospital Reimbursement. By 1948, the Blue Cross Commission and the AHA's new council promoted a single package of hospital and medical benefits, along with nationwide coverage for large employers.

Bugbee saw three principal functions for the AHA: standards and research, education, and advocacy. "They so feather together than you can hardly tell which is which," he told his successor, Edwin L. Crosby, M.D., in a 1959 conversation. Bugbee thrived on hospital management—his goal was a bookshelf of manuals serving as essential references for hospital administrators. He and his staff went a long way toward filling the shelf, publishing a series of manuals on such topics as admitting practices, managing insurance claims, purchasing supplies, and the use of radioisotopes.

Also in the 1940s, the AHA formed an educational trust to accept tax-deductible gifts and grants for research and education aimed at improving hospital care. The Commission on Hospital Care and its nationwide survey was the trust's first project. This arm of the AHA was later renamed the Hospital Research and Educational Trust, and more recently the Health Research and Educational Trust.

With support from the Kellogg Foundation, the AHA and the trust created the Commission on Financing of Hospital Care, which focused much of its agenda on the health care problems

Managed Care Is Born
Industrialist Henry Kaiser (left) and Sidney Garfield., M.D., attend the dedication of Kaiser Permanente's Oakland Hospital in 1942. Kaiser founded the HMO giant the same year, inspired in part by Garfield's work in developing health services for migrant construction crews in the West.

Source: Kaiser Permanente

of the elderly. The commission was headed by Arthur C. Bachmeyer, M.D., a hospital administrator and University of Chicago professor who had served as AHA president in 1926. Its findings, released during the Eisenhower administration, helped build momentum for Medicare.

Interest in better patient care led to a string of initiatives and commissions during the 1940s and '50s. These activities raised the AHA's profile and increased its influence on national health policy. The association teamed up with the AMA, the American Nurses Association, the National League for Nursing, the American Public Health Association, and the American Public Welfare Association to raise professional and institutional standards and improve care for the chronically ill. The AHA also became a key participant in the Joint Council to Improve the Health Care of the Aged, another group laying the groundwork for Medicare.

Growth and change also continued inside the AHA. To include governing boards more formally in the policy structure, the association founded a section for hospital trustees and began publishing *Trustee*, a monthly magazine. The AHA also urged greater involvement of women in health care, supported volunteers in hospitals, and organized its own Committee on Women's Hospital Auxiliaries, which ultimately evolved into the Committee on Volunteers. It entered the 1950s with a new mission: "To promote the public welfare through the development of better hospital care for all the people."

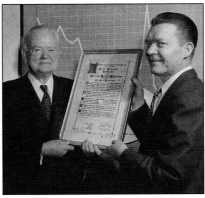

A Citation from Hoover
Former President Herbert Hoover, chairing a citizen's advisory panel in 1956, cites the AHA and its Blue Cross Commission for aiding public welfare. Ray Brown, the AHA's top elected member, receives the honor. The link with Blue Cross was dissolved a decade later.

Source: Tommy Weber

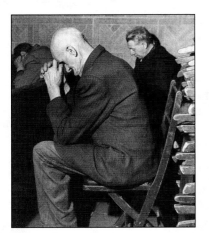

Making the Case for Medicare
As the health care troubles of the elderly repeatedly rose to the surface, the AHA's Eisenhower-era Commission on Financing of Hospital Care pressed the case for a nationwide response.

Source: Hulton Getty/Tony Stone Worldwide

Times change, but some themes play out again and again. When Edwin Crosby became the AHA's top executive in 1954, Capitol Hill was assailing hospitals for rising costs and spiraling services. Crosby contended that the field was being attacked unfairly by politicians and government officials. "No institution in the United States has received more challenges to change than has the hospital," he told the AHA House of Delegates. "Buffeted from all sides, hospitals are asked to provide the most costly of treatment facilities and then are criticized for the expense of treatment."

Like Bugbee, Crosby was uncomfortable with Washington politics and avoided the confrontations typical of congressional hearings on Capitol Hill. He appointed his deputy director, Kenneth Williamson, to head the new Washington office. Among his duties, Williamson represented the interests of hospitals on 26 provisions of the Medicare and Medicaid statute. When he left after 18 years, he was succeeded by Leo J. Gehrig, M.D., a retired official of the U.S. Navy and Public Health Service.

Not long after Crosby arrived, the AHA staff outgrew its Chicago headquarters on Division Street. In 1957 the House of Delegates authorized a four-year, 100 percent dues surcharge to finance a new building at 840 North Lake Shore Drive. Chicago

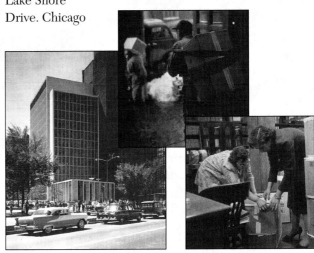

A Lakefront Home
A four-year, 100 percent hike in dues helped finance new headquarters on Chicago's Lake Shore Drive, with groundbreaking in 1959. Ten years later, the AHA added a west building with a connecting link. Source: Grant Jacoby Studios

Mayor Richard J. Daley was among the groundbreakers in January 1959.

Ten years later, the association added a west building, with a connecting link to its existing home. Tenants included the American College of Hospital Administrators, the American Protestant Hospital Association, and the Blue Cross Association.

The scope of AHA activities broadened again in the 1960s. Leaps in diagnosis and treatment included kidney and heart transplants and the proliferation of intensive care units. From the mid-1950s to the mid-'60s, the number of hospital employees doubled nationally. Social and political reform led to the Civil Rights Act of 1964, the enactment of Medicare, and other pieces of President Lyndon Johnson's Great Society.

At the AHA, staff experts in virtually every area of hospital management worked with member committees, issued advisories, and answered phone calls and letters from anyone working or volunteering at member hospitals. George Bugbee's dream for the AHA came true—and then some. Its staff and councils produced dozens of manuals, monographs, periodicals, and issue papers on insurance, staffing, areawide planning, health care data, community relations, disaster preparedness, and other issues of the day. The AHA also kept up its role in setting standards for the field. In 1963, it joined the American Association of Medical Record Librarians in recommending use of the International Classification of Diseases as a coding system.

AHA membership expanded again, bringing Blue Cross plans, hospital schools of nursing, and areawide planning agencies to the rolls. The association reorganized personal membership in 1962, setting up societies to improve the skills of hospital managers. The American Society for Hospital Engineering was the first personal membership group.

On the national front, the AHA supported Medicare in principle, but with some reservations. Fewer than half of elderly Americans had health insurance when Medicare came on the scene. The needy aged "should be eligible on an insurance basis for free health ser-

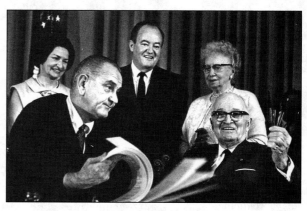

At Long Last—Medicare
Harry Truman never saw his view of compulsary national health insurance made the law of the land, but he lived to see the advent of Medicare and Medicaid. President Johnson flew to Truman's home in Independence, Mo., for the 1965 signing ceremony. Source: AP/Worldwide Photos

vices," an AHA official statement said. "The program should afford assistance to as many of the aged as practicable, without regard to their individual financial resources in purchasing health insurance on a reasonable contributory basis."

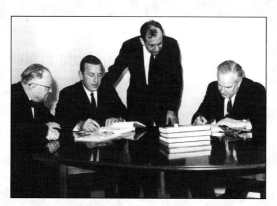

Administering Medicare
AHA chief Edwin Crosby (left) looks on as Blue Cross president Walter McNerney signs a pact making Blue Cross a fiscal agent for Medicare. Social Security chief Robert Ball (right) signs his copy under the eye of Arthur Hess, head of the Bureau of Health Insurance.

Source: Blue Cross/Blue Shield

Largely in response to Medicare and other federal changes, the AHA took a hard look at its own programs and services. A committee chaired by John H. Knowles, M.D., director of Massachusetts General Hospital, made more than 50 recommendations, including a broader base of financing. The committee suggested a separate study of the interlocking board relationship with the Blue Cross Association, a move that eventually led to dissolving that arrangement. "It was necessary for them to separate, not because they were too close, but because their relationship was perceived that way," said prepayment expert Robert Sigmond.

Thanks to Medicare, commercial insurance, and hundreds of federal and state regulations, the field had grown complex and diverse. Needing to better organize grassroots policy and advocacy work, the AHA turned to state and metropolitan hospital associations to create the Partnership for Action in 1968. Largely under the leadership of Washington office chief Leo Gehrig, the part-

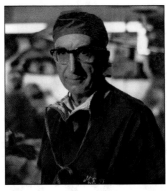

Leaps in Medicine
Heart surgery pioneer Michael DeBakey of Baylor College of Medicine remains a symbol of major strides in medicine during the '60s and '70s.

Source: William R. Pittman

nership gave the AHA the ability to act on legislative proposals and policy matters. It also set up nine geographic boards to enhance policy deliberations. The Regional Advisory Boards—which consisted of members of the House of Delegates and executives from the state and metropolitan associations—began meeting regularly.

Two years later, the AHA strengthened its grassroots emphasis when it held the first annual membership meeting in Washington to create a policy forum and organize lobbying for executives from hospitals and state and metropolitan associations. The attendance list has always included congressional leaders with a stake in health care legislation, federal health officials, health care leaders, and journalists. Presidents Nixon and Clinton have addressed the meeting; during the 1984 session, AHA officials met with President Reagan at the White House.

Near the end of the 1960s, the AHA took its boldest steps yet into health policy. The Special Committee on the Provision of Health Services, popularly known as the Perloff Committee, called for Ameriplan, a restructuring of delivery and financing "to make health care more accessible, more comprehensive, more responsive, and more relevant to the needs of the community." Along with chairman Earl Perloff, board chairman of the Albert Einstein Medical Center and Philadelphia General Hospital, the 15-member group included three doctors, two health lawyers, a member of the clergy, and six hospital administrators. Alex McMahon, the association's president from 1972 to 1986, still calls it "a proposal way ahead of its time."

Ameriplan's centerpiece was the health care corporation, an organization charged with pro-

viding a complete range of care for people in its geographic area. Each corporation would cross political boundaries when necessary to ensure that everyone had access to care. "It was a forerunner of today's integrated delivery systems and the current emphasis on community health," said Perloff committee member Edward J. Connors, who served as AHA chairman in 1989. "Many changes in health care networking that parallel developments of the 1990s were embodied in Ameriplan."

But AHA members sharply disagreed over Ameriplan. Some saw it as an invitation to the government bureaucracy it professed to avoid, while others feared its sweeping overhaul of the system. The AHA House of Delegates approved Ameriplan conceptually in January 1971 and several months later approved a policy statement on providing health

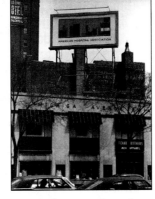

National Hospital Week, 1967
With federal health regulation an increasingly potent force, the AHA became more visible on the policy scene and in the public eye.

services, which was drawn from Ameriplan. The AHA also endorsed basic provisions of a congressional bill substantially based on Ameriplan and introduced by former Rep. Al Ullman (D-Ore.), then the #2 Democrat on the House Ways and Means Committee.

Talk of major structural reform led the AHA to look at other basics. In 1969 and 1970, a committee developed the association's first statement on health care for the disadvantaged, but its work was far more sweeping. The statement held members accountable for all health care needs in their communities and described hospitals as central resources that must relate to all care providers and to all environmental, governmental, and social agencies in their regions. It also talked about the role of hospitals in preventing disease; maintaining and restoring health; improving services for the disadvantaged; and involving consumers in their health care decisions.

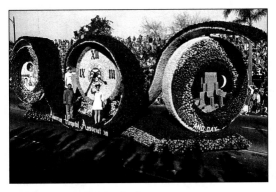

Caring 'Round the Clock
The AHA's 1972 float in the Tournament of Roses Parade came at a time of heightened concern for the disadvantaged. That led to the first Patient's Bill of Rights, adopted in 1973 and revised in 1992. Source: Chicago Photographers, Inc.

"Though more people are better served by hospitals now than in the early 1970s, many of the principles enunciated by the committee remain at the heart of the AHA's vision for healthier communities," said H. Robert Cathcart, a chair of the Committee on Health Care for the Disadvantaged and AHA chairman in 1976. Not surprisingly, the committee also created the landmark Patient's Bill of Rights, which the AHA approved in 1973. That document stood unchanged until 1992, when it was revised by a panel on biomedical ethics.

In February 1972, following a national search, the AHA Board of Trustees appointed North Carolina Blue Cross executive John Alexander McMahon as the first president, the top staff position. At that time, the title of the AHA's elected leadership position was changed from president to chairman. Arriving in the midst of congressional concern over hospital costs and growing Medicare outlays, McMahon sought to strengthen the AHA's visibility in Washington. Hospitals had already had a year of federal price controls under the Nixon administration's economic stabilization program; rarely had the association been so challenged.

Under McMahon, the AHA became embroiled in high-profile advocacy in defense of the field's interests. The AHA's concerns about rising hospital costs and the

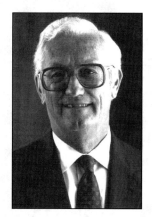

Alex McMahon, 1972
His 14-year term as AHA president was marked by a fight against federal payment caps and greater visibility on Capitol Hill.

government's arbitrary attempts to control them peaked during the decade. In his 1976 report to the House of Delegates, McMahon vowed to "fight with every means at my command" President Ford's proposed cap on Medicare payments to hospitals, which the AHA believed would force members to cut services. McMahon's commitment to oppose caps on payments also dominated AHA advocacy through the Carter administration.

At the height of the Carter cap turmoil, the association rose to a challenge by Rep. Dan Rostenkowski (D-Ill.) to voluntarily control spending or suffer the consequences of government control. With the AMA and the Federation of American Hospitals (now the Federation of American Health Systems), the AHA organized the Voluntary Effort, aimed at reducing the rate of increase of community hospital expenses by 2 percent in both 1978 and 1979. The effort met with much cynicism. Yet within a year, the groups documented lower hospital spending and showed that percentage increases in the gross national product and in hospital expenditures from March 1978 to March 1979 were identical. The AHA's persistent opposition helped defeat President Carter's cost containment bill. Not long after, costs began to climb again, though more slowly. But the Voluntary Effort's most significant victory was in unifying doctors and hospitals.

A Mission in Motion: Words Change, but Basics Remain

The association's first members set out to exchange ideas on the nitty-gritty of running hospitals. In doing that, they launched hospital management as a profession. The founders also put the mission of hospitals squarely on the side of patients and their communities. That remains fundamental today. In its centennial year, the AHA still flies the banner of community health improvement.

The evolution of the AHA's mission over the past 100 years hints at major shifts in both health care and American society. These few words, revised and amended at various points for various reasons, show how the hospitals have perceived themselves and their role in the midst of technological, clinical, and policy changes.

1899: "To facilitate the interchange of ideas, comparing and contrasting methods of management, the discussion of hospital economics, the inspection of hospitals, suggestions of better plans for operating them, and such other matters as may affect the general interest of the membership."

1907: "The object of this association shall be promotion of economy and efficiency in hospital management."

1917: "To promote the welfare of the people so far as it may be done by the institution, care and management of hospitals and dispensaries with efficiency and economy; to aid in procuring the cooperation of all organizations with aim and object similar to those of this association; and, in general, to do all things which may best promote hospital efficiency."

Throughout the 1970s, the AHA continued to focus on the problems of access to care and financing. It appointed an advisory panel to consider alternatives, including regulation of health care institutions as public utilities and state review of hospital rates. The House of Delegates even voted to propose federal legislation for national standards and guidelines for state rate review. But that position wasn't long-lived, since support for rate regulation proved shallow once the threat of more onerous measures decreased.

AHA advocacy increasingly called attention to the conflict between demands for quality care and cost control. As national health insurance again became a major issue, the association urged that any plan for universal health insurance combine cost containment with ways to moderate demand. It used the term "universal" rather than "national" to emphasize coverage for everyone versus a monolithic federal program. A landmark AHA document, a revision of the 1969 Statement on the Financial Requirements of Health Care Institutions and Services, declared that all purchasers of health care must recognize and "share fully" in the total financial requirements of hospitals.

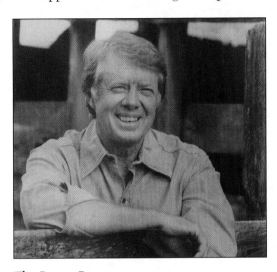

The Carter Caps
Cost concerns, smoldering for years in Congress, became red hot during the Carter presidency. The AHA took up a challenge from former Rep. Dan Rostenkowski to rein in expenses or face federal caps—a campaign known as the Voluntary Effort.
Source: AP/Worldwide Photos

As the association increasingly acted as both a defender of hospital interests and an advocate of broader public values, it sought to better understand the dichotomy. A committee—led by John M. Stagl, then president of Chicago's Northwestern Memorial Hospital and the association's chairman in 1977—declared that the AHA is both a trade group and a public interest organization, a distinction that underscored increasing involvement in national health policy. In 1978, the AHA formed a political action committee to increase its effectiveness in Washington.

As the association looked for new ways to balance heavy demands for health care with cost control, it turned to the business community. By 1985, more than 130 business and health coalitions had formed nationwide, and McMahon saw the need to work with business leaders on cost-effective solutions. He began meeting with these coalitions. Nationally, the AHA

1938: "To promote the welfare of the people through the development of hospital and outpatient service. To further this object the association shall encourage professional education and scientific research, aid in the health education of the public, cooperate with other organizations having a similar object, and do all things which may best promote hospital and outpatient service efficiency."

1951: "To promote the public welfare through the development of better hospital care for all the people."

1973: "To promote the welfare of the public through its leadership and its assistance to its members in the provision of better health care and services for all the people."

1987: "Its mission shall be to promote high-quality health care and health services for all the people through leadership in the development of public policy, leadership in the representation and advocacy of hospital and health care organization interests, and leadership in the provision of services to assist hospitals and health care organizations in meeting the health care needs of their communities."

1995: "The mission of AHA is to advance the health of individuals and communities. AHA leads, represents, and serves health care provider organizations that are accountable to the community and committed to health improvement." ⌒

became part of a group of health, labor, and business leaders who studied health care issues under the leadership of John Dunlop, a professor at Harvard University and former U.S. labor secretary.

Also in the late 1970s, the AHA stepped up its interest in an emerging force known as managed care. Executive vice-president Gail L. Warden—who went on to become CEO of Detroit's Henry Ford Health System and AHA chairman in 1995—led discussions on HMOs, capitation, and related issues, frequently echoing concepts inherent in the Perloff report. "Forces outside the structure of the hospital field started to change 30 years ago when the Commission on the Cost of Hospital Care talked about the hospital being the center for community health," Warden said recently. "Now we're seeing the reality, as hospitals are viewed as major social institutions, adding value to their communities."

Warden was also the architect of the AHA's constituency centers, which focus on the needs of multihospital systems as well as rural and urban hospitals. In response to a shortage of nurses, the AHA, the Hospital Research and Educational Trust, and American Hospital Supply Corp. sponsored the National Commission on Nursing. Participants included the American Nurses' Association, the National League for Nursing, the AMA, the American Association of Colleges of Nursing, and academics. Its far-reaching recommendations spoke to nursing practice, education, and the public role in licensing and educational funding.

The field's changing insurance needs led the AHA to form two subsidiaries in the 1970s: AHA Insurance

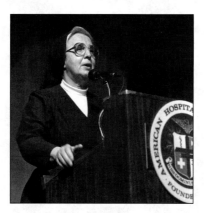

Sister Irene Kraus, 1980
The first woman to chair the AHA Board of Trustees, she urged consumers and hospital trustees to get more involved in health affairs. She also held no-nonsense views about running hospitals. "No margin, no mission," she often told audiences.

Source: Chad Evans Wyatt

Carol McCarthy, 1986
In her five years at the helm, the AHA pressed for Medicare changes that did not simply slash payments to doctors and hospitals.

Source: Chad Evans Wyatt

Resource, which now serves the insurance, financial, and information needs of providers, and the Health Providers Insurance Co., a malpractice reinsurance company later sold in 1995.

McMahon affirmed the increasingly accepted view—for decades rejected by many hospital administrators—that governing boards should become more involved in the public arena, along with doctors and hospital executives. This position was strengthened officially by the AHA's Committee on Hospital Governing Boards in its 1975 report and at the 1979 AHA Conference on Hospital Governance. At the conference, Sister Irene Kraus, former president of the Daughters of Charity National Health System and AHA chairman in 1980, told the audience to expect much more involvement from both trustees and consumers in health affairs. At the same time, the AHA insisted that the public had unmet responsibilities and should better understand its role in holding down costs and eliminating unnecessary and costly government regulations.

With Medicare costs continuing to sound alarms in Congress, the association's Council on Finance recommended prospective pricing and diagnosis-related groups to control and better predict Medicare spending. After much debate, in 1982 the House of Delegates lent its support to PPS, and the AHA lobbied Congress to enact the system. AHA members continued to raise concerns about the system's fairness, a dominant theme of the association's policy deliberations. The association reconciled dozens of implications—geographic payment differences, wage issues, case mix adjustments, and socioeconomic differences among patients—first through its policymaking and then through advocacy.

At the same time, the field was growing increasingly alarmed about the effect of reductions in Medicaid and other programs that represent a safety net for the poor. The Special Committee on Federal Funding of Mental Health and Other Health Services (more popularly known as the Kinzer Committee after its chairman, David M. Kinzer, then president of the Massachusetts Hospital Association) produced a report, *Health Care: What Happens to People When Government Cuts Back*. It galvanized the association's policy and strategy on Medicaid and other coverage issues. Discussions about the report also led to policy strategies to address care for the medically indigent. Most were later incorporated into the AHA's proposal for overhauling the health care system.

The 1980s also brought new threats from infectious diseases to all hospitals. In a report laying out a hospitalwide approach to AIDS, the AHA dealt not only with patient safety and confidentiality, but also the safety of staff, personnel management, and public relations. In response to the growing bioethical dilemmas facing the membership, particularly in terms of life-sustaining care decisions, the association convened a committee of ethicists, administrators, nurses, and doctors to develop guidance.

In the early 1980s, a board committee headed by 1983 chairman E. E. Gilbertson took another look inward. The committee said the AHA should focus on hospitals and health systems as its primary institutional members and increase the voice of major constituencies in its policy structure. The constituency centers became "sections," with governing councils and seats in the House of Delegates. The association's council structure was refined, trustees became further involved, and multihospital systems received greater say in policy and governance. The AHA also recognized the influential role of nurse executives, leading to the establishment of the American Organization of Nurse Executives as an AHA subsidiary.

In 1986, when Carol M. McCarthy, Ph.D., succeeded McMahon as president, the association was deeply involved in debates over the future of Medicare and Medicaid. Steadily rising federal outlays continued to stir debate in Congress. Most Capitol Hill proposals were aimed at providers rather than beneficiaries, the least politically risky approach. Throughout McCarthy's five years at the AHA, she battled changes that the AHA argued would threaten the quality of patient care and hospital solvency.

Association leaders increasingly saw that the existing payment system inevitably was ratcheting down payments year by year, and they began calling for fundamental changes. The Board of Trustees started work on health care reform principles that later guided the AHA through national debates in the early 1990s. "It was a big change for the association," said McCarthy, "particularly

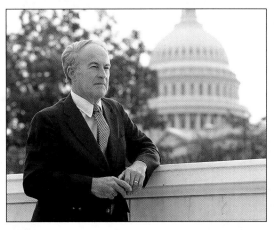

Policy Veteran
Jack Owen, who ran the Washington office from 1982 to 1991, became interim president after McCarthy resigned. He continued work on the AHA's principles for long-term health care reform, a task began by McCarthy.

in having to craft policies that might not protect the continuation of every one of its members in their existing structures."

Growing competition, mergers, and other shifts in the market began to dominate discussions about the field's future. At the same time, the AHA began to analyze its own role with an eye to streamlining operations and making participation more feasible for busy executives. The AHA standing councils were replaced by ad hoc committees that could complete their work on sharply focused issues in six months or a year. The Regional Advisory Boards became Regional Policy Boards. The Board of Trustees also set up an Institutional Practices Committee to oversee management guidance materials.

During McCarthy's stint as president, the AHA began rethinking its programs and services, a process that continues under the presidency of her successor, Dick Davidson. "It was and is a sign of the times," McCarthy said recently. "Associations are truly being challenged today to do more with less for a different type of member." When McCarthy left the AHA, Jack W. Owen, who had been director of the Washington office since 1982, was named acting president. Owen, a

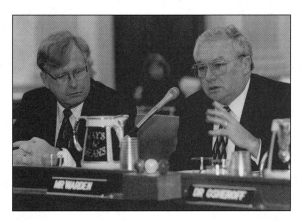

Policy Voice
Members are the experts: That's the founding principle of today's AHA advocacy and services. Gail Warden, CEO of Henry Ford Health System in Detroit and AHA chairman in 1995, lays out the AHA's position in testimony to Congress. Source: Bill Fitz-Patrick

veteran of Medicare wars on Capitol Hill, was instrumental in the association's growing involvement in government payment policy.

The 1990s have brought the most sweeping changes ever to hospitals, the AHA, and all of health care. Organizations are merging, consolidating, acquiring, or being acquired more rapidly than at any other time in the nation's history. Along with advances in medical technology, the integration of services is having a profound effect.

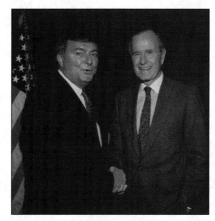

Dick Davidson
Since he took the AHA's top job in 1991, the Office of the President moved to Washington to boost lobbying. He also has led a major rethinking of programs and services.

Dick Davidson, longtime CEO of the Maryland Hospital Association, became AHA president in 1991, bringing new philosophies on how an association should relate to its members and other groups. Rather than mobilizing a cadre of management experts, Davidson viewed the association's role as providing forums for member interaction, best practices, and colleague-to-colleague learning. He viewed members as participants in advocacy and representation and added venues for grassroots education and lobbying by the members. Davidson also strengthened partnerships with state associations in both policy and advocacy. With health care reform clearly on the national agenda, he moved the Office of the President to Washington so that the AHA had a more visible and accessible presence. A streamlined Chicago staff moved into more modern offices in the Loop.

The board's work at refining its health reform principles continued, with Davidson urging a critical look at the organization of the health care system. The result was a plan that puts patients first and calls for partnerships with doctors, other health professional groups, business, government, labor, insurers, schools, and the public. The AHA's Community Care Network℠ concept focuses on

providing a full range of services, community accountability, a health status focus, and payment via capitation. "It allows us to get back to our roots and return the patient to the center of our health care system," said Carolyn Roberts, the AHA's 1994 chair. Although President Clinton's overhaul of health care failed, the AHA's concept of integrated care focused on community health status continues to guide its advocacy on incremental reform and public health.

"AHA members are excited that their association is for something that represents true health care reform, a plan that is driven by community-based values," Davidson said. "It takes us away from the perverse incentives of fee-for-service medicine to managing health care in the community and emphasizes prevention." He pointed out that many of its provisions are already occurring in the field without legislative or regulatory action. Community

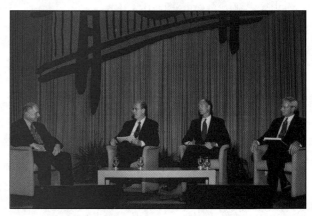

Pacesetters, 1995
Consultant Gerry McManis (left) leads a panel pondering trends in the field at the San Francisco convention: Gordon Sprenger, executive at Allina Health System and AHA chairman in 1996; Richard Scott, former CEO of Columbia/HCA; and Richard Neeson of Independence Blue Cross. Source: Oscar and Associates

---

Community Care Network, Inc. uses the name Community Care Network as its service mark and reserves all rights.

care networks are under way in many states, evident in the National Community Care Network Demonstration Program cosponsored by the AHA, the Health Research and Educational Trust, the Catholic Health Association, and VHA, an alliance of not-for-profit hospitals.

It was a small step from this view to the AHA's new vision and mission based on community health and adopted in 1995: "The AHA vision is of a society of healthy communities, where all individuals reach their highest potential for health. The AHA mission is to advance the health of individuals and communities. AHA leads, represents, and serves health care provider organizations that are accountable to the community and committed to health improvement."

In 1996 and '97, the board and the strategic planning committee began reshaping the AHA to serve its changing membership in the next century. With the focus on the vision and mission, they aim to open up the AHA to new members, while keeping a strong emphasis on hospitals and systems. They're considering ways to make dues more equitable and link advocacy and services to the new vision. Changes in governance and policymaking—and even the name itself—will be on the table during the 1998 centennial year.

With health insurance still a national concern, the AHA has embarked on a two-year Campaign for Coverage to reduce the number of Americans without health insurance by 10 percent—4 million people—within two years. The campaign draws on the work of state and metropolitan associations and commitments from members.

At the same time, the AHA has taken steps to restore public trust in the health care system. For 20 years, opinion polls have reflected the view that health care institutions are focused more on business needs than on patients and communities, an impression strengthened in the last year by the federal government's efforts to define

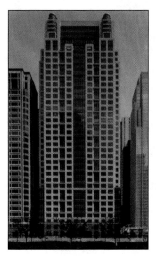

View from the Loop
The AHA left its outdated Lake Shore Drive headquarters in 1994, moving its streamlined staff to One North Franklin in Chicago's Loop.

Medicare billing errors as fraud and abuse violations. The AHA has urged its members to adopt regulatory compliance programs to minimize errors and better conform to complicated federal rules.

On the merger and acquisition front, the association has developed guidelines for changes in hospital ownership that recommend detailed accountability to communities. The AHA also is sponsoring public opinion research and emphasizing patient involvement in decisionmaking as an important element of quality of care.

"The field has never lost its values of caring for people and trying to do a better job," Davidson said recently. "The AHA has always felt a sense of accountability to communities." He's optimistic about what this means for the future, "when health care organizations compete and collaborate at the same time." Among his goals—based on his family's experience since he became AHA president—is better treatment of patients at the end of life. "We have a long way to go, as we better integrate and coordinate care. And I hope we can help to make some inroads."

Davidson sees incremental change—such as recent legislation expanding coverage for uninsured children—as the clear path for further reform of the health care system. "Incremental change has been our history in health care, and now we're beginning to see change on that very basis," he said. "It's certainly evident in expanded choice under Medicare and in efforts to maintain choice in the workplace."

Whatever unfolds at whatever rate, the AHA's vision puts the association in a good position for growth and member advocacy, Davidson added. "Our mission dates from that first evening in Cleveland 100 years ago when a small group of hospital superintendents thought it was a good idea to get together. As history tells us, it was. And now we have an opportunity that none of us would want to miss." ☞

Elected Presidents and Chairs of The American Hospital Association

1899–2000

1899	James S. Knowles	Lakeside Hospital	Cleveland, OH
1900	James S. Knowles	Lakeside Hospital	Cleveland, OH
1901	Charles S. Howell	Western Pennsylvania Hospital	Pittsburgh, PA
1902	Jesse T. Duryea, M.D.	Kings County Hospital	Brooklyn, NY
1903	John H. Fehrenbatch	Cincinnati General Hospital	Cincinnati, OH
1904	Daniel D. Test	Pennsylvania Hospital	Philadelphia, PA
1905	George H. M. Rowe, M.D.	Boston City Hospital	Boston, MA
1906	George P. Ludlam	New York Hospital	New York, NY
1907	Renwick R. Ross, M.D.	Buffalo General Hospital	Buffalo, NY
1908	Sigismund S. Goldwater, M.D.	Mount Sinai Hospital	New York, NY
1909	John M. Peters, M.D.	Rhode Island Hospital	Providence, RI
1910	H. B. Howard, M.D.	Peter Bent Brigham Hospital	Boston, MA
1911	W. L. Babcock, M.D.	Grace Hospital	Detroit, MI
1912	Henry M. Hurd, M.D.	Johns Hopkins Hospital	Baltimore, MD
1913	Frederic A. Washburn, M.D.	Massachusetts General Hospital	Boston, MA
1914	Thomas Howell, M.D.	New York Hospital	New York, NY
1915	William O. Mann, M.D.	Massachusetts Homeopathic Hospital	Boston, MA
1916	Winford H. Smith, M.D.	Johns Hopkins Hospital	Baltimore, MD
1917	Robert J. Wilson, M.D.	Willard Parker Hospital	New York, NY
1918	Arthur B. Ancker, M.D.	City and County Hospital	St. Paul, MN
1919	Andrew R. Warner, M.D.	Lakeside Hospital	Cleveland, OH
1920	Joseph B. Howland, M.D.	Peter Bent Brigham Hospital	Boston, MA
1921	Louis B. Baldwin, M.D.	University Hospital	Minneapolis, MN
1922	George O'Hanlon, M.D.	Bellevue Hospital	New York, NY
1923	Asa S. Bacon	Presbyterian Hospital	Chicago, IL
1924	Malcolm T. MacEachern, M.D.	American College of Surgeons	Chicago, Il
1925	E. S. Gilmore	Wesley Memorial Hospital	Chicago, IL
1926	Arthur C. Bachmeyer, M.D.	Cincinnati General Hospital	Cincinnati, OH
1927	R. G. Brodrick, M.D.	Alameda County Hospital	Oakland, CA
1928	Joseph C. Doane, M.D.	Philadelphia General Hospital	Philadelphia, PA
1929	Louis H. Burlingham, M.D.	Barnes Hospital	St. Louis, MO
1930	Christopher G. Parnall, M.D.	Rochester General Hospital	Rochester, NY
1931	Lewis A. Sexton, M.D.	Hartford Hospital	Hartford, CT
1932	Paul H. Fesler	Wesley Memorial Hospital	Chicago, IL
1933	George F. Stephens, M.D.	Winnipeg General Hospital	Winnipeg, Man., Can
1934	Nathaniel W. Faxon, M.D.	Strong Memorial Hospital	Rochester, NY
1935	Robert Jolly	Memorial Hospital	Houston, TX
1936	Robin C. Buerki, M.D.	State of Wisconsin General Hospital	Madison, WI
1937	Claude W. Munger, M.D.	St. Luke's Hospital	New York, NY
1938	Robert E. Neff	State University of Iowa Hospitals	Iowa City, IA
1939	G. Harvey Agnew, M.D.	Canadian Medical Association	Toronto, Can
1940	Fred G. Carter, M.D.	St. Luke's Hospital	Cleveland, OH
1941	B. W. Black, M.D.	Alameda County Institutions	Oakland, CA
1942	Basil C. MacLean, M.D.	Strong Memorial Hospital	Rochester, NY
1943	James A. Hamilton	New Haven Hospital	New Haven, CT
1944	Frank J. Walter	St. Luke's Hospital	Denver, CO

1945	Donald C. Smelzer, M.D.	Germantown Dispensary and Hospital	Philadelphia, PA
1946	Peter D. Ward, M.D.	Charles T. Miller Hospital	St. Paul, MN
1947	John H. Hayes	Lenox Hill Hospital	New York, NY
1948	Graham L. Davis	W. K. Kellogg Foundation	Battle Creek, MI
1949	Joseph G. Norby	Columbia Hospital	Milwaukee, WI
1950	John N. Hatfield	Pennsylvania Hospital	Philadelphia, PA
1951	Charles F. Wilinsky, M.D.	Beth Israel Hospital	Boston, MA
1952	Anthony J. J. Rourke, M.D.	Hospital Council of Greater New York	New York, NY
1953	Edwin L. Crosby, M.D.	Joint Commission on Accred of Hospitals	Chicago, IL
1954	Ritz E. Heerman	California Hospital	Los Angeles, CA
1955	Frank R. Bradley, M.D.	Barnes Hospital	St. Louis, MO
1956	Ray E. Brown	University of Chicago Clinics	Chicago, IL
1957	Albert W. Snoke, M.D.	Grace-New Haven Community Hospital	New Haven, CT
1958	Tol Terrell	Shannon West Texas Memorial Hospital	San Angelo, TX
1959	Ray Amberg	University of Minnesota Hospitals	Minneapolis, MN
1960	Russell A. Nelson, M.D.	Johns Hopkins Hospital	Baltimore, MD
1961	Frank S. Groner	Baptist Memorial Hospital	Memphis, TN
1962	Jack Masur, M.D.	National Institutes of Health	Bethesda, MD
1963	T. Stewart Hamilton, M.D.	Hartford Hospital	Hartford, CT
1964	Stanley A. Ferguson	University Hospitals of Cleveland	Cleveland, OH
1965	Clarence E. Wonnacott	Hosp Syst of Church of Jesus Christ LDS	Salt Lake City, UT
1966	Philip D. Bonnet, M.D.	Univ. Hospital, Boston Univ. Med Center	Boston, MA
1967	George E. Cartmill	Harper Hospital	Detroit, MI
1968	David B. Wilson, M.D.	University Hospital	Jackson, MS
1969	George W. Graham, M.D.	Ellis Hospital	Schenectady, NY
1970	Mark Berke	Mount Zion Hospital and Medical Center	San Francisco, CA
1971	Jack A. L. Hahn	Methodist Hospital of Indiana	Indianaplis, IN
1972	Stephen M. Morris	Samaritan Health Service	Phoenix, AZ
1973	John W. Kauffman	Princeton Hospital	Princeton, NJ
1974	Horace M. Cardwell	Memorial Hospital	Lufkin, TX
1975	Wade Mountz	Norton-Children's Hospital	Louisville, KY
1976	H. Robert Cathcart	Pennsylvania Hospital	Philadelphia, PA
1977	John M. Stagl	Northwestern Memorial Hospital	Chicago, IL
1978	Samuel J. Tibbitts	Lutheran Hosp. Soc of Southern California	Los Angeles, CA
1979	W. Daniel Barker	Crawford W. Long Mem Hosp of Emory Univ	Atlanta, GA
1980	Sister Irene Kraus	Providence Hospital	Washington, DC
1981	Bernard J. Lachner	Evanston Hospital	Evanston, IL
1982	Stanley R. Nelson	Henry Ford Hospital	Detroit, MI
1983	E. E. Gilbertson	St. Luke's Regional Medical Center	Boise, ID
1984	Thomas R. Matherlee	Gaston Memorial Hospital	Gastonia, NC
1985	Jack A. Skarupa	Greenville Hospital System	Greenville, SC
1986	Scott S. Parker	Intermountain Health Care	Salt Lake City, UT
1987	Donald C. Wegmiller	HealthOne Corp.	Minneapolis, MN
1988	Eugene W. Arnett	Memorial Hospital of Taylor County	Medford, WI
1989	Edward J. Connors	Mercy Health Services	Farmington Hills, MI
1990	David A. Reed	Samaritan Health Services	Phoenix, AZ
1991	C. Thomas Smith	Yale-New Haven Hospital	New Haven, CT
1992	D. Kirk Oglesby, Jr.	Anderson Area Medical Center	Anderson, SC
1993	Larry L. Mathis	The Methodist Hospital System	Houston, TX
1994	Carolyn C. Roberts	Copley Hospital	Morrisville, VT
1995	Gail L. Warden	Henry Ford Health System	Detroit, MI
1996	Gordon M. Sprenger	Allina Health System	Minneapolis, MN
1997	Reginald M. Ballantyne III	PMH Health Resources, Inc.	Phoenix, AZ
1998	John G. King	Legacy Health System	Portland, OR
1999	Fred L. Brown	BJC Health System	St. Louis, MO
2000	Carolyn B. Lewis	Greater Southeast Health System	Washington, DC

INDEX

National Alliance for the Mentally Ill
(NAMI), 73
National Association of Children's
Hospitals and Related Institutions, 95
National Association of Public Hospitals
& Health Systems (NAPH), 47
National Commission on Nursing, 112
National Community Care Network
Demonstration Program, 115
National health policy, 111
National Health Service bill, 106
National Hospice Association (NHO), 97
National Hospital Association (NHA), 19
National Hospital Record, 103
National Hospital Week, 109
National Information Center for Health
Services Administration, 103, 104
National Institutes of Health
(NIH), 16–17
National Labor Relations Act (1935), 54
National Labor Relations Board, 55
National Medical Association (NMA), 19
National Museum of Civil War
Medicine, 2, 3
National Organ Transplantation
Act (1984), 35
National Vaccine Injury Compensation
Program (1986), 39
Native Americans, epidemics
among, 92–93
Neeson, Richard, 114
Neonatology, 79
Nevins, David, 7
New Deal, 64–65
AHA and, 105
Social Security and, 52
New England Medical Center, 45, 95
New York Children's Hospital, 94
New York City almshouse, 46, 47
New York Infirmary for Women and
Children, 101
Nightingale, Florence, 10–11, 80
NIH. *See* National Institutes of
Health (NIH)
911, 7
Nixon, Richard, HMOs and, 50, 51
North Carolina, health care for rural resi-
dents in, 58–59
Northridge earthquake, 63
Northwestern Memorial Hospital
(Chicago), 105
Nosocomial infections, 89
Nuns. *See* Catholic nuns
Nurses and nursing, 10–11, 112
AIDS and, 74–75
careers and, 105–106
male nurses, 75
Nursing services, 45
Nutrition, 80–81

Occupational therapy, 5
Office of Indian Affairs (OIA), 92–93
Ohio Hospital Association, 104
Operating rooms, asepsis in, 89
Organ transplants, 34–35. *See also* Clark,
Barney
ORYX policy, 31
Owen, Jack W., 113–114

Paget, Stephen, 36
Pancreas transplants, 35
Paramedics, 7
Pariseau, (Mother) Joseph, 61
Partnerships, of AHA, 114
Pasteur, Louis, 88, 89
Patients, postcards from, 68, 69
Patient's Bill of Rights, 110
Pediatrics, 95
neonatology and, 79
Pennsylvania Hospital of
Philadelphia, 42, 98
Pension coverage, 25
Perloff Committee, 109
Pertussis, 39
PET. *See* Positron emission tomography
(PET)
Pharmacy, 98–99
Philadelphia, children's health care in, 94
Philadelphia College of Pharmacy, 99
Philadelphia Hospital, 4–5
Philanthropists, 42–43
Physick, Phillip Syng, 5
Polio, 26–27, 39
Political action committee, 111
Politics, 107. *See also* Legislation;
Lobbying
Pop culture, perspective on health
care, 20–21
Popovich, Rose, 101
Positron emission tomography (PET), 67
Postcards, from patients, 68, 69
Post-polio syndrome, 27
Post-traumatic stress disorder, 71
Poverty, medical care during Great
Depression, 64
PPS, 112
Premature babies, 78–79
Presidents and chairs, of AHA, 116–117
Prospective pricing, 112
Prosthetic devices, 70–71
Provident Hospital and Training
School, 19
Publications, of AHA, 103
Public health
Great Depression and, 64–65
influenza pandemic and, 13
philanthropies and, 43
Public Health Service, 57, 85
Public Health Service Act (1944), 17
Public hospitals, 46–47

Public policy, 112
AHA and, 103, 109
national health policy and, 111
Public welfare, 107
Pure Food Laws, 33

Quinlan, Karen Ann, 48–49

Racial discrimination, AHA and, 102
Red Cross, 86
Reed, Walter, 85
Reform, of medical education, 22–23
Regional Advisory Boards, 109, 113
Regulation, by Food and Drug
Administration, 32, 33
Rehabilitation, 70–71
Rehabilitation Institute of Chicago, 77
Research
NIH and, 16–17
by VA, 70–71
Respiratory distress syndrome, 78, 79
Restoration work, 70–71
Revolutionary War, hospitals
during, 84–85
Richardson, Katharine, 94
Rights. *See* Civil rights
Roberts, Carolyn, 114
Roberts, Elliott C., Sr., 19
Roberts, Jonathan, 98–99
Rockefeller Foundation, 42, 43
Roentgen, Wilhelm, 66
Roosevelt, Franklin D. *See also*
Great Depression
health care reform and, 52
polio and, 27
Rorem, C. Rufus, 104
Rosenberg, Charles, 95
Rostenkowski, Dan, 110
Rural health care, 58–59
Rush, Benjamin, 5
Rutkow, Ira M., 82, 83

Sabin, Albert, 27
St. Elsewhere (television program), 21
St. Mary's Hospital for Children
(Bayside, NY), 95
Salk, Jonas, 27
Salk vaccine, 38, 39
Saltonstall, William, 44
San Francisco earthquake, 62–63
Saunders, Cicely, 96–97
Schwartz, Steven, 21
Scott, Richard, 114
Segregation, hospitals and, 19
Semmelweis, Ignac, 88–89
Shellshock, 71
Sigmond, Robert, 108
Sisters of Charity of the Incarnate
Word, 60–61
Slaves and slavery, hospitals for
blacks and, 19